Practical English *for* Dental Technology

2nd edition

Practical English *for* Dental Technology

2nd edition

[저 자]
최 병 환
박 미 영

[감 수]
James Parr

대한나래출판사

Preface

이 책은 치과기공에 사용되는 전문용어 숙지 및 치과와 거래 시 발생하는 다양한 상황에서 필요한 영어를 적절하게 구사하는 데 그 목적을 두고 있다. 또한 해외의 치과기공소나 치과 재료 개발 및 해외 시장 마케팅을 주 업무로 하는 치과 재료업체 취업 준비생을 위한 교과서로 활용될 수 있을 것이다. 나아가 해외 취업을 준비하는 경력 기공사는 물론 해외 치과와 거래하는 우리나라 기공소 담당자를 위한 지침서로서의 활용도 가능할 것이다. 다소 난이도 높은 표현이 있으나 전체적으로 치과기공 교육 이수자의 수준에 맞추어 기술하였다.

"Practical English for Dental Technology" 제2판은 총 13 Chapter로 구성되어 있다. 각 Chapter는 해외에서 일어나는 상황에 적절히 대응할 수 있는 기본적인 일반 회화와 치과기공과 관련한 특정 주제로 구성되어 있다. 활용의 편의를 위해 크게 3개의 섹션으로 구분하였다. Chapter 1~7에서는 치과기공 관련 일반 회화 중심으로, Chapter 8~11은 치과기공물 제작 과정을, 마지막으로 무역 관련 용어와 회화가 Chapter 12~13에 담겨져 있다. 제2판에서는 각 단원마다 미국 실생활에 맞춘 생존 영어를 추가하였다.

한 번 더 언급하면 치과기공 관련 영어에 대한 지식이 부족한 학생들에게 전문용어를 소개함과 동시에, 최고의 기술을 구비하고도 해외 취업 시 취약했던 언어 문제의 해소를 통한 글로벌 마인드 정립과 자신감 고취를 위한 것이다. 또한 우리나라와 다른 해외 기공 문화와 제 규정 등에 대한 정보의 부족으로 부진하였던 해외 기공물 수출업의 영업력 향상에 밑거름이 되고자 한다.

처음 출간되는 이 책은 '치과기공 관련 전문용어 및 회화'라는 측면에 중점을 두었다. 책을 엮은이는 치기공 전공자와 영어 전공자이며, 원어민 교수에게 감수를 받아 꼭 필요한 전공 분야의 용어 및 회화를 현지 생활 언어에 맞춰 구성하여 각 주제에 관련된 용어를 연습해 나가다 보면 어느새 자연스럽게 영어로 말하는 자신의 모습을 발견하게 될 것이다.

바라건대 본 교재가 영어에 대한 자신감을 갖고 세계 최고의 치과기공사로서 대한민국 치과기공기술을 널리 전파하는 데 일조할 수 있기를 바란다.

2015년 8월

대구보건대학교 영송관에서

최 영 환

Contents

Chapter 1

Entry & Leave

1. 공항에서 (공항, 기내, 입출국)

Key expressions

1. At Airport

1) Departure

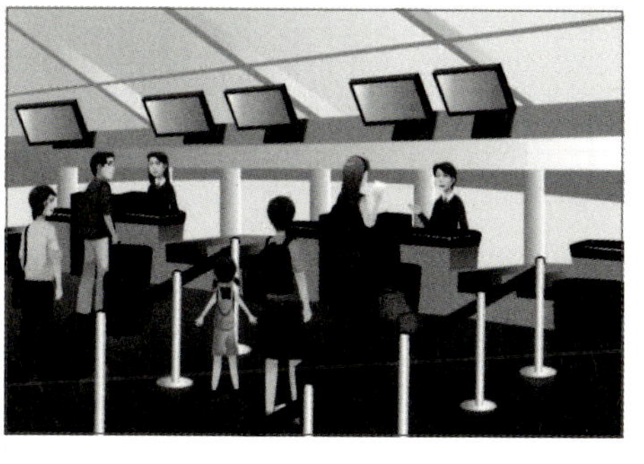

A : Would you prefer window or aisle seat?

B : I prefer window seat / aisle seat.

A : Your bags are overweight, you need to something out or pay an extra charge.

B : I will pay an extra charge. / OK. I will check it now.

2) Arrival

A : Where can I pick up my baggage?

B : What was your flight number?

A : I was on UA 7000.

B : Your baggage is on carousel #3.

A : I think I lost my baggage.

B : Can I see your baggage claim ticket?

A : Here it is.

2. At Cabin

1) Take off

Good afternoon, welcome aboard. This is your Captain Jenny Choi.
Our Flying time to Seattle will be 10 hours and 30 minutes after take-off.

Local time on the ground is now 1:50, so you might like to adjust your watches.

Temperature at our destination is 19 degrees Celsius or 66 degrees Fahrenheit,
and skies are clear with a slight breeze,
although some rains are predicted for earlier this morning.

In about another 40 minutes, after we reach our cruising altitude of 22,000 feet,
refreshments and a light brunch will be served.

Later our flight attendants will distribute our in-flight catalog of duty free goods.

Please take a minute to familiarize yourself
with the information regarding this aircraft and emergency procedures,
which you can find on the card in the seat pouch in front of you.

Please make sure that your seat belt is securely fastened
and retrain from smoking during the entire flight.
Also, the use of portable electronic devices is not allowed during take-off and landing.
For your comfort and safety,
all heavy or fragile items must be placed under the seat in front of you.
Once we are airborne,
I have turned off the seatbelt sign, and you are free to move about the cabin.
However, I strongly recommend that you remain seated
with your seatbelt fastened when the seatbelt sign is on.

Passengers are reminded once again that this is non-smoking flight.

If there is anything we can do to help make your flight more comfortable,
please don't hesitate to ask.

2) Landing

The plane will touch down at the airport soon.
Connecting passengers will be advised flights when we reach our destination.
Before leaving the aircraft,
please check to make sure that you have not left any belongings.

Thank you for flying with our DaehanNarae Air,
and we wish you have a pleasant stay here in Seattle.

Unit

- Tc(℃) = temperature in degrees Celsius
- Tf(°F) = temperature in degrees Fahrenheit
- Tc = (5/9)*(Tf − 32)
- Tf = (9/5)*(Tc + 32)
- 1 feet = 30.48 centimeter
- 1 gallon = 3.78 liter
- 1 pound = 0.45 kilogram

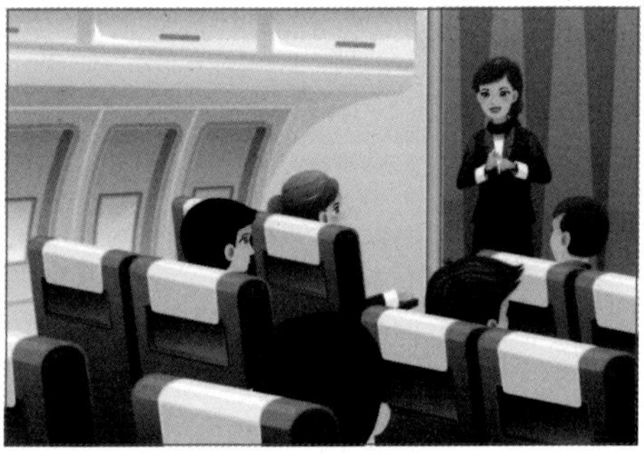

A : What would you like, chicken or beef?

B : Chicken please. / Beef please.

A : What would you like to drink?

B : What do you have? Do you have coke?

Can I get some water? / more blanket?

A : Please fasten your seat belt.

Please put your seat forward

Sign

- VACANT
- OCCUPIED
- RETURN TO SEAT
- NO CIGARETTE DISPOSAL
- FLUSH TOILET
- HAND TOWELS ONLY
- SHAVER OUTLET

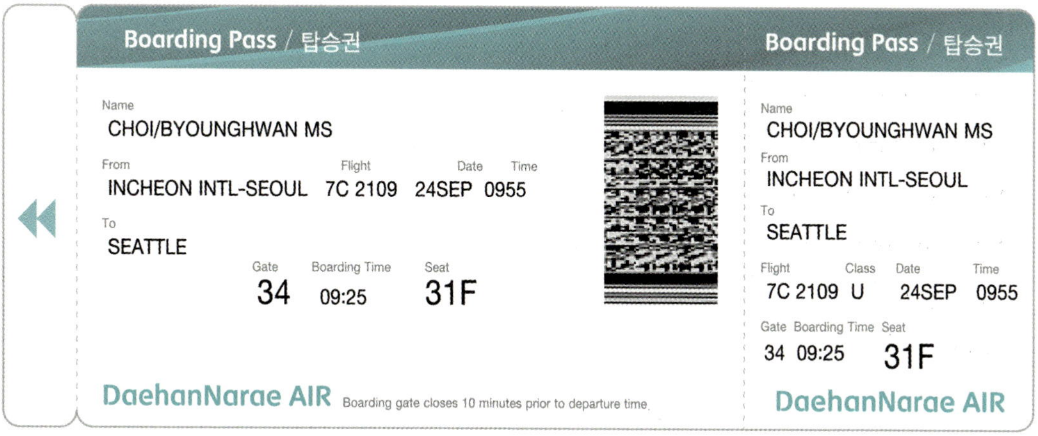
Boarding Pass / 탑승권
Name
CHOI/BYOUNGHWAN MS
From
INCHEON INTL-SEOUL
Flight
7C 2109
Date
24SEP
Time
0955
To
SEATTLE
Gate
34
Boarding Time
09:25
Seat
31F
DaehanNarae AIR
Boarding gate closes 10 minutes prior to departure time.
Boarding Pass / 탑승권
Name
CHOI/BYOUNGHWAN MS
From
INCHEON INTL-SEOUL
To
SEATTLE
Flight Class Date Time
7C 2109 U 24SEP 0955
Gate Boarding Time Seat
34 09:25 31F
DaehanNarae AIR

3. At Immigration

A : Your passport and immigration card please.

B : OK. Here it is.

A : What is the purpose of your visit?

B : I am here on business. / for trip.

A : How long will you be staying in the U.S.?

B : For two months.

A : Where will you be staying?

B : I will be staying in hotel.

A : Do you have anything to declare?

B : Yes / No.

Vocabulary

- **Aisle seat** : A seat next to a path (passageway)
- **Extra charge** : Additional payment
- **Carousel** : A moving surface from which passengers can collect their luggage
- **Fasten your seat belt** : Tie up seat belt
- **Put your seat forward** : Do not make your seat backward
- **Passport** : Official document containing your name, photograph, and personal details, which you need to show when you enter or leave a country
- **Immigration card** : The paper which you should notify to the office about your entry status
- **Declare** : You say how much you have bought or earned so that you can pay tax on it

2. 외국인의 학교 방문 시 안내

School visitors

A : Welcome to Korea, and of course welcome to our school.
Hope you are not jet lagged too badly.
My name is Jenny.
For the next 3 hours, I will be your guide around the school.
May I ask where you are from?

B : I am from New jersey, USA.
Are you a student of dental technology?

A : Yes. I am.
Are you a dentist or a dental lab technician?

B : I am an owner of Fine Art Dental Lab.

A : Good! so you can understand me.
Let's begin our tour without further delay.
This is an eight-story building.
Our department uses the first to fourth floors.
As you can see to your right, this is a laboratory for partial dentures.
2nd year students are practicing in this room.
All appliances are equipped for practice.

B : What year are you in?

A : I am a second year student.

B : What courses are you taking this semester?

A : I'm taking Complete Dentures, Fixed Prosthodontics, Removable Partial Dentures, Principles of Occlusion, Dental Ceramics, Orthodontics, and Dental Materials.

3. 치기공과 소개

Department of Dental Technology

Tooth Morphology

A study of tooth shape, structure and function; drawings of 28 permanent teeth and deciduous teeth, wax buildup of the anatomical crowns for maxillary and mandibular teeth.

Complete Dentures

A removable prosthesis that replaces all teeth on the mandibular arch or on the maxillary arch supported by the surrounding soft and hard tissues.

Fabricating impression trays, constructing baseplates and wax occlusal rims, articulating casts, setups, wax-ups, flasking, wax elimination, packing, deflasking, selective grinding, finishing and polishing, and repairs.

Fixed Prosthodontics

Fixed prosthesis is the replacement of missing teeth with a prosthesis permanently cemented in place. Such Restorations include; crowns, bridges (fixed dentures), veneers, fixed implant restorations, inlays and onlays. Construction of casts and dies, identifying margins, trimming and ditching dies, articulation, developing wax patterns, investing, casting, finishing and polishing of single-unit or multi-unit restorations.

Crown : Crowns are referred to as 'caps' and completely cover all surfaces of a natural tooth. Crowns can be fabricated from many different materials such as gold, composite resin, ceramic.

Bridge : Bridges are fabricated to restore gaps between natural teeth (conventional) or on just one side (cantilever).

Inlay : Inlay is fitted to a cavity in a small amount of missing tooth and cemented into place. The inlay can be made from metals, resins, ceramics, amalgam and composite.

Onlay : An onlay is similar to an inlay, but it covers over the cusps of a tooth.

Veneer : Veneer is a thin layer of ceramic or resin that is placed onto the surface of a tooth to restore damaged teeth, rotated teeth, or to improve esthetics.

Dental Ceramics

1 cl hr, 6 lab hrs, 24 hrs externship, 4 cr (spring only)

Dental ceramic (also known as dental porcelain) is a ceramo-metal dental restoration and all-ceramic restoration. Design and construction of metal copings (frameworks), investing and casting of non-precious metals, pre-soldering and post-soldering of non-precious metals, application and firing of opaques, contouring and firing of porcelains and glazing and staining, finishing and polishing. During the summer, externship students will be placed in dental lab to gain real world exposure.

Removable Partial Dentures

Removable restorations that replace one or more teeth and remain stable in normal function but can be removed by the patient for cleaning and at night. Surveying, designing, duplicating the master casts, wax-up and casting, finishing and polishing of metal frameworks, arranging teeth, waxing, flasking, packing, deflasking, finishing and polishing of acrylic.

Science of Dental Metallurgy

The study of dental metallurgy, physical and mechanical properties of metals, their internal structure and types of precious and nonprecious dental casting alloys and metals used in the laboratory.

Computer Aided Design/Computer Aided Manufacturing (CAD/CAM) in Dentistry

CAD/CAM dentistry is the theory and practice of fabricating dental prosthetics digitally to improve the design and creation of dental restorations, especially dental prostheses including crowns, veneers, inlays and onlays, fixed bridges, dental implant restorations, dentures (removable or fixed), and orthodontic appliances.

CAD/CAM : Scanning and designing dental models from digital impressions.

Orthodontics

Orthodontics is concerned with the study and treatment of malocclusions, which may be a result of tooth irregularity and disproportionate jaw relationships. Orthodontic appliances are made with wires, springs and screws to move teeth and form a more harmonious occlusion and esthetic appearance of teeth or to maintain the position of previously moved teeth.

Fixed Prosthodontics Practicum

A practical techniques and procedures learned in the basic courses. Actual impressions are used in all restorative dental cases in the classroom.

Prerequisite : Completion of all third level courses

Required courses

- *Semester I* (11 units)

Denture Techniques (4.0 units)

Crown and Bridge (4.0 units)

Dental Morphology (0.5 units)

Beginning Dental Anatomy (1.5 units)

Directed Studies in Basic Dental Laboratory Techniques (1.0 units)

&

- *Winter intersession first year* (2.5 units)

Intermediate Dental Anatomy (1.5 units)

Directed Studies in Intermediate Dental Laboratory Techniques (1.0 units)

&

- *Semester II* (13.5 units)

Dental Materials (2.0 units)

Denture Techniques (4.0 units)

Crown and Bridge (4.0 units)

Advanced Dental Anatomy (2.5 units)

Directed Studies in Advanced Dental Laboratory Techniques (1.0 units)

&

- *Semester III* (13.5 units)

Highly Advanced Dental Anatomy (2.5 units)

Orthodontics and Pedodontics (2.0 units)

Ceramics (4.0 units)

Partial Dentures (4.0 units)

Directed Studies in Basic Dental Laboratory Techniques (1.0 units)

&

- ***Winter intersession second year*** (4.5 units)

  Clinical Experience (3.5 units)

  Directed Studies in Intermediate Dental Laboratory Techniques (1.0 units)

  &

- ***Semester IV*** (13 units)

  Advanced Ceramics (6.0 units)

  Partial Dentures (2.0 units)

  Dental Laboratory Management (2.0 units)

  Transition to Dental Laboratory Industry (2.0 units)

  Directed Studies in Advanced Dental Laboratory Techniques (1.0 units)

- ***Required electives*** (5 units)

  or

- ***Additional required courses***

  General Education Common Core (20 credits)

  Required Core (3 or 4 courses, 11-14 credits)

  English Composition (1 or 2 courses, 3 or 6 credits)

  (http://www.citytech.cuny.edu/academics/catalog_listing.shtml)

Chapter 2

Introduce

1. 소개/인터뷰하기

Key expressions

1. Self-introduction

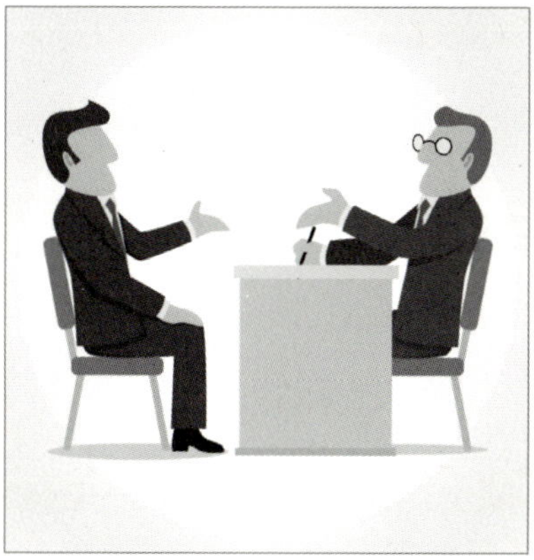

A : Please make a brief introduction about yourself.

B : I am very happy to introduce myself to you. My name is Jae-seok and I graduated from Daegu Health College in dental technology in 2014.

I have many of relevant experiences, including a 3-month internship last year with dental laboratory.

I could learn variety of techniques related to dental technology and dealing with affairs also.

That was valuable experiences for me which would be useful for this position with your company.

Working here has been my career objective since I was a junior in college.

I really want to pursue a career with your organization.

Thank you.

2. Interview

A : What do you do weekends?

B : I enjoy living a balanced life between work and rest.

So in my free time, I often enjoy playing soccer in a local soccer league.

A : What are your strength and weakness?

B : I think honesty is my trademark.

I always live and work honestly.

I never mix company business with my personal interest.

On the other hand, I have excessive desire for maximum performance of tasks which is distributed to me.

And it could make other colleagues tired.

So I think that is my weakness.

A : Do you have any skills or licenses?

B : I have dental technician license and I can make dentures, braces and implants.

A : How do you make people accept your idea?

B : I usually communicate effectively with others to resolve conflicts.

A : Why do you want to work for this company?

B : Your company always has been ranked the best dental technical laboratory to work for.

Also my personality is well-matched to your company and I have a number of strengths to offer your company.

Vocabulary

- **Dental technology** : A skill of making dental appliances
- **Dental technical laboratory** : A company which makes dental appliances
- **Affairs** : Business, tasks, an event
- **Honesty** : Marked by truth, frank
- **Task** : Any piece of work that is undertaken, a specific piece of work required to be done
- **Excessive** : Beyond normal limits
- **Distribute** : Give as in small portions
- **Personality** : Which can characterize a unique individual

2. 면접 예상 질문

Job interview questions

- What are your strengths and weaknesses?

- Describe your work style.

- What are your career goals and where do you see yourself in the next 5 years?

- Tell me why you want to work here.

- What type of work environment do you prefer?

- Describe your best boss and your worst boss.

- What kinds of people do you find it difficult to work with?

  ex) People who lie, people who blame others, someone who doesn't work hard

- Do you prefer to work alone or on a team?

- What makes you unique from other candidates?

- How would you assess your communication skills?

  ex) In terms of English communications skills I might not have a best skills but I think I'm a good listener and someone who tries to understand others.

- Why did you choose your major or area of work?

- How would your professor or past supervisors describe you?

  ex) I think they would tell you that I'm a hard worker, and that I work well on a team.

- What can you do for our company?

- Have you ever had difficulty working with a colleague?

- What did you like or dislike about your previous job?

- Have you gotten angry at work? What happened?

- How do you handle pressure?

- How long do you expect to work for this company?

- How much do you expect to get paid?

- Why should we hire you and not other people?

- Is there anything else I can tell you about the job and the company? / Do you have any questions about our company or this position?

3. 이력서 작성

Resume writing

Cover letter template

Cover Letter에 포함되어야 하는 사항

- 첫 번째 페이지의 오른쪽 위에 이름, 이메일 주소와 전화번호 입력
- 왼쪽에 지원 회사명과 담당자 이름 입력
- 오른쪽에 작성 날짜 입력
- 참고사항(예 : "Re : 포세린 파트 지원")
- 담당자에게 인사(예 : "Dear Mr.Choi", "To whom it may concern"는 사용하지 말 것)
- 자신의 간략한 소개글 작성
- 지원한 파트와 관련된 경력이나 기술을 강조하여 작성
- 입사를 간절히 원한다는 내용으로 마무리

Cover letter sample

Jenny Choi

Email : ilovehwani95@hanmail.net

Mobile : XXX XXXX XXXX

Mr Inho Jang

Minchul Kim and Associates

Phone : XX XXXX XXXX

Email : jih@adl.com

07 May 2015

RE : Application for Plaster work

Dear Mr. Jang,

As a motivated individual I am extremely interested in submitting an application for the advertised Plaster Work position.

In February 2013 I graduated from Daegu Health College, Department of Dental Technology. This has given me practical capabilities that will meet the needs of this role.

While completing college courses I worked part-time as a Plaster Work Assistant for Elite Dental Lab. My responsibilities in this role included construction of casts and dies, articulation, investing, and casting. This work has given me practical job skills, allowing me to experience working in a professional and fast-paced work environment.

My professors and employers have praised me for my high level of ability and friendly personality. I want to learn new things and I enjoy both challenges and meeting objectives. Please feel free to contact my current and previous supervisors.

I realize this job opening will have lots of competition. However, I believe my commitment and skills will allow me to make a positive contribution to your organization.

I would appreciate the chance to meet with you to go over my application. Enclosed is a copy of my resume. Please contact me at any time if you need further information.

Thank you for your consideration.

Jenny Choi

Sample resume format

이름

현주소

원주소

전화번호(cell, work, home phone number)

- **희망 직종(career objective)** : 25글자나 그보다 짧게 명확한 목표 설정을 해서 강한 동기를 가지고 그 업무를 담당할 충분한 마음의 준비가 되었다는 것을 구인 측에 나타낼 수 있도록 작성. 어떤 직종을 희망하는지를 우선적으로 첫 부분에 명시

  예 : Entry level position in Plaster Work. Long-range goal CAD/CAM Technician.

- **교육(education)** : 졸업 연도와 전공과목을 포함하여 최종 학력부터 작성

- **자격증(certification)** : 보유하고 있는 모든 자격증 작성

- **특기(specialized skills)** : 지원자의 특기 사항 입력(CAD design, computer 등)

- **근무 경력(employment history or work experience)** : 실습, 시간제 아르바이트를 포함하여 최근 경력부터 모두 작성

- **수상 경력(honors, leadership, and awards)** : 직업과 관련된 장학금을 포함하여 모든 수상 경력 작성

- **추천서(References)** : 지원자의 자질이나 능력을 확인할 수 있는 사람의 연락처와 이름을 명시. "References available upon request"

Sample resume

Jenny Choi

email : xxx@xxx.com

PRESENT ADDRESS :
850 BeomMul-Dong,
SuSeong-Gu, Daegu,
South Korea

PERMANENT ADDRESS
314 DaeMyung-Dong, Buk-Gu,
Pohang, Gyeongbuk,
South korea
Phone# : (+82)10-xxxx-xxxx

OBJECTIVE Entry level position in Plaster Work. Long-range goal Ceramist and CAD/CAN designer

EDUCATION Daegu Health College, Daegu, South Korea February 2013
Intended Major : Dental Technology

EXPERIENCE **Digital Dental Laboratory, Daegu, South Korea, Feb, 2013-Present**
Construction of casts and dies, trimming and ditching dies, articulation, investing, casting and polishing

High Dental Laboratory, Daegu, South Korea, June - Aug, 2012
Completed a rigorous externship

EZ Dental Laboratory, Daegu, South Korea, Dec, 2011 - Feb, 2012
Completed a rigorous externship

SKILLS	• Computer skills :		
	Power Point	CAD/CAM system	Microsoft Office 2000
	Microsoft Excel	Microsoft Access	Adobe PhotoShop 5.0
AWARDS	Won 'Presentation Competition' hosted by Daegu Health College 2011		
CERTIFICATE	iBT 110, 2012.10		
ACTIVITIES	Volunteered at Dong-Daegu welfare center (100 hrs.)		
REFERENCES	Available upon request		

Chapter 3

Office

1. 회사에서 (휴가, 봉급, 승진, 사직, 해고 등)

Key expressions

1. Daily routine

A : Good morning. How are you?

B : I am busy. I have three meetings today.

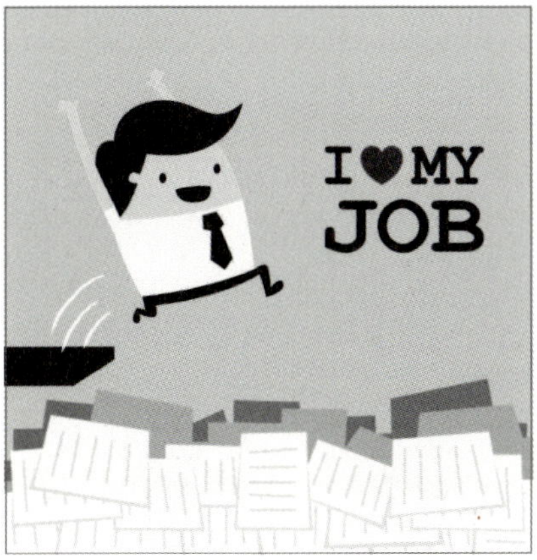

A : Would you help me with this report?

B : Sorry, we are already understaffed due to the ongoing project.
We are behind schedule.
We are pressed for time.

A : Please go over the first draft on the report.

B : OK. I'll check it. But if you need more data, refer to the report for the last year.

A : Oh, thank you. I need to wrap it up for today.

2. Holiday / Vacation

A : I need to get away from it all.

A : Where will you go for vacation?

B : I will go to Hawaii.

A : How long will you be gone?

B : About a week.

A : Who should I contact about the tasks you did?

B : Mr. Kim will cover for me.

3. Salary

A : The season for salary negotiation is around the corner.

A : Based on my current salary, I was expecting something within the 3 to 4,000 range.

A : OK. I will take it. / I would like to accept your offer.

4. Promotion

A : I heard you got promotion recently. Congratulations!

B : Yeah, I was promoted to branch chief. Thank you.

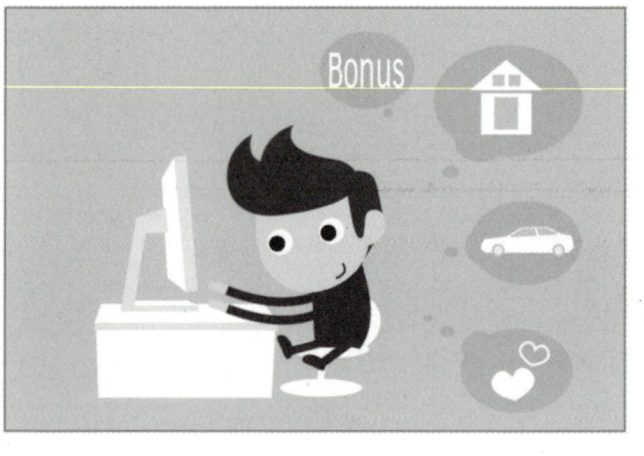

5. Resignation & Dismissal

A : I have been offered a better job. So unfortunately I need to quit here.

A : This letter is to give formal notice of my intention to leave the company, effective Jun 29, 2014.

A : The company notified the labor union of the dismissal of seventy employees.

A : He was fired and is now out of work.
B : I am sorry to hear that.

6. Retirement

A : He announced his retirement from his position.
B : Yeah, He really worked very hard during thirty years.

Vocabulary

- **Understaffed** : Inadequate in number of workers or assistants, lack of workers
- **Behind schedule** : Late, left unfinished
- **Wrap up** : Finish a task completely
- **Get away** : Remove oneself from a familiar environment usually for pleasure
- **Salary** : Pay, wage
- **Negotiation** : A discussion intended to produce an agreement
- **Promote** : Assign to a higher position
- **Resignation** : The act of giving up, your intention to resign
- **Dismissal** : Official notice that you have been fired from your job
- **Fired** : Having lost your job
- **Retirement** : withdrawal from your position or occupation

2. 기공사 소개

Dental technicians

Dental technicians construct custom made restorations and dental appliances upon prescription from a dentist. They work in specialties including crowns and bridges, complete dentures, partial dentures, orthodontic appliances and ceramics.

Dental technicians communicate with the dentists with prescriptions, drawings and measurements taken from patients. A dental impression is the most important thing that the technicians flow a gypsum dental stone to construct of the patients anatomy known as a dental cast. Technicians use this cast for the construction of custom prosthesis.

There are three major parts within dental technology. These are removable prosthesis, including full dentures and partial dentures; fixed prosthesis including crowns, bridges, inlay, implants; and orthodontics, including orthodontic appliances and mouth guards.

Employment facts

Dental technicians held more than 39,000 jobs in 2012. They generally work full time in small laboratories, but some work in laboratories that employ hundreds of technicians.

Educational requirements

Some colleges and technical schools offer formal educational programs, but most people receive only on-the-job training. At first, one will learn how to do simple tasks like pouring plaster into an impression, and later on he or she will learn how to make dental prosthesis.

Other requirements

Although it is not required some dental technicians want to become certified. The National Board for Certification established by the National Association of Dental Laboratories, offers certification which is based on experience and an exam.

3. 해외 면허증

CDT (Certified Dental Technology)

CDT는 면허증이 아닌 자격증으로 NBC(National Board for Certification)의 관리하에 운영되고 있으며 ceramics(CE), crown & bridge(CB), partial dentures(PD), complete denture(CD), ortho-dontics(OD), 그리고 Implants의 6과목으로 이론과 실습을 통해 취득할 수 있다.

자격

학교(2 years) 졸업 + 2년 경력 또는 5년 이상의 경력자

※ 한국에서 4년제를 졸업하였다 하더라도 2년만 인정

The Comprehensive and Recognized Graduate Examinations (공통, 2시간 45분)

160문항(written multiple-choice test, 실제 시험에는 10문제 추가되지만 정답만 성적에 포함됨)

- 과목 – History, ethics and the six specialties (oral anatomy, tooth morphology, materials science, health & safety, fundamental theory and terminology)

The written specialty exam (1시간 30분)

- 시험 과목 – Ceramics, Complete Dentures, Crown & Bridge, Orthodontics, Partial Dentures and Implants.
- 80문항 (multiple-choice questions, 10문제 추가)

Practical Examination (5시간 30분)

- Hands-on exam
- 시험 당일 도착 – 7:00 am
- 시작 – 7:50 am

Contents

Removable Prosthodontics-Complete Dentures

- 상악 custom tray 제작
- 28개의 인공치 배열
- 치은 형성
- 2개의 의치 수리(인공치 교체, 파절된 의치 수리)
- 상악 baseplate와 wax rim 제작

Removable Prosthodontics-Partial Dentures

- 상악과 하악의 Survey와 framework design, 복제모형 준비
- Wrought wire clasp를 연결한 framework 미리 준비
- 상악과 하악 복제모형에 디자인을 바탕으로 wax up
- 미리 준비한 metal framework를 연마

Fixed Prosthodontics-Crown & Bridge

- 3본 브릿지 wax up
- 나뉜 3본 브릿지를 solder 후 연마
- MOD 케이스를 wax 후 연마

Fixed Prosthodontics-Ceramics

- 준비해 온 금속 coping 다듬질
- Coping에 porcelain butt margin 완성
- Opaque 도포 후 도재 완성
- 여분의 coping wax

Orthodontics

- Hawley-type의 장치물 완성
- 가철식 하악 편측 sagittal 장치물 완성
- 고정식 하악 lingual arch 완성

Implants

- 2개의 치아를 각각 diagnostic wax up
- Matrix와 screw retained custom abutment와 substructure 제작
- Verification jig 제작
- Hader Bar attachment를 이용하여 하부 구조물 제작
- 14개의 치아 set up과 wax up

Application Process and Fees

지원자는 아래 웹 주소를 방문하여 CDT Handbook과 Application을 클릭 후 원서를 작성하면 된다. Handbook에는 CDT가 되기 위한 절차와 방법 등 필요한 모든 정보가 제공되어 있다.

(https://nbccert.org/certificants/certified-dental-technician/)

- CDT Comprehensive Exam: $220
- CDT Specialty Written Exam: $220
- CDT Practical Exam: $455*

※ $55(non-refundable)이 추가된 금액이다.

CDT 시험 일시 공지

https://nbccert.org/education/exam-finder/NBC-pdf-cdt-exam-calendar.cfm 참조

Application for Certified Dental Technician
All CDT Examinations

For Office Use Only:	Candidate# ______________
Received ______________	Site# ______________
Approved ______________	Date ______________

I. APPLICANT INFORMATION

1. Name ______________ Dr./Mr./Mrs./Ms./Miss/Other ______

2. CDT (if adding a specialty or reinstating) or RG # (if applicable) ______________

3. Street Address ______________

____

City ______________ State ______________ Zip ______________

4. E-mail ______________ 5. Work Phone ______________

6. Home or Cell Phone ______________ 7. FAX ______________

8. Date of Birth ______________

II. EXAM SELECTION

1. I hereby apply for certification testing in the specialty of dental laboratory technology indicated below. Please check next to the specialty in which you will be testing. Only one specialty may be selected.

☐ Complete Dentures ☐ Partial Dentures ☐ Crown & Bridge ☐ Ceramics ☐ Orthodontics

You will be signed up for the Comprehensive exam, the Written Specialty exam in the area indicated above and the Practical exam in the same specialty.

2. Preferred examination location and date, selected from the current examination schedule on www.nbccert.org. Applications may not be accepted after the deadline specified for each exam without NBC approval and a late fee of $100 ($25 per written exam and $50 for the Practical exam).

First Choice: City ______________ Date ______________

Second Choice: City ______________ Date ______________

Applicants for exams are accepted in the order they are received by the NBC Headquarters up to the capacity of each facility. If your first choice location is filled, you will be contacted and assigned, if possible, to your second choice location. If the NBC cannot accommodate you at either your first choice or your second choice location, you are entitled to a refund of your examination fee or you may have your application and fees held until a location becomes available for you.

III. LANGUAGE REQUIREMENT

Do you read, speak and write the English language? ☐ Yes ☐ No

IV. LEGAL REQUIREMENT

Have you been convicted of illegal practice of dentistry? ☐ Yes ☐ No

V. EDUCATION

1. Did you graduate from high school or the equivalent (such as earning a GED)? ☐ Yes ☐ No
2. List post-secondary studies and degree(s) earned, if any:

Name of Institution	Courses or Major	Degree Earned	Year of Graduation

VI. APPLICANT'S CURRENT EMPLOYMENT

1. Present Employer_______________
2. Business Address_______________

____

City _______________ State _______________ Zip _______________

3. Date of Employment _______________ ☐ Full-time ☐ Part-time (hrs. per week_____)
4. Name and title of present supervisor _______________
5. Brief description of the work you do _______________

____

____

6. Are you responsible for supervising the performance of other technicians or production personnel on a daily basis? ☐ Yes ☐ No
7. Are you regularly or occasionally responsible for the instruction or training of other technicians?
☐ Yes ☐ No

continued...

All Certified Dental Technician Examinations Application, continued.

VII. APPLICANT'S PREVIOUS EMPLOYMENT

The NBC requires that CDT applicants have at least five years of education and/or employment in dental technology, unless the applicant is a Registered Graduate (see Eligibility for CDT Certification Exams). You must supply such information as the NBC might need to verify compliance with this requirement — including the complete mailing addresses and names of employers and supervisors. This requirement is interpreted to mean five (5) years of full-time employment (at least 35 hours per week) and additional credit is not awarded for formal education concurrent with employment claimed towards this requirement.

1. Most Recent Employer ____________________

   Business Address ____________________

   ____

   City ____________ State ____________ Zip ____________

   Telephone: ____________

   a. Dates employed:

   from (month and year) ____________ until (month and year) ____________

   ☐ Full-time ☐ Part-time (hrs. per week_____)

   b. Job title and brief description of duties performed ____________

   ____

   ____

   ____

   c. Name of Supervisor ____________________

2. Employment prior to position listed above ____________________

   Business Address ____________________

   ____

   City ____________ State ____________ Zip ____________

   Telephone: ____________

   a. Dates employed:

   from (month and year) ____________ until (month and year) ____________

   ☐ Full-time ☐ Part-time (hrs. per week_____)

   b. Job title and brief description of duties performed ____________

   ____

   ____

   ____

   c. Name of Supervisor ____________________

Please use additional pages if needed to report at least five years of dental technology training, education and experience.

VIII. ATTESTING SIGNATURES

You, as a CDT applicant, must obtain attesting signatures from two persons — *who are current Certified Dental Technicians or licensed dentists* — who believe that you demonstrate competence in the dental technology specialty for which you seek certification.

To the attesting persons: Your signature below testifies that you are familiar with the skills and abilities of this CDT applicant, and that you are satisfied with the applicant's competence to fill dental prescriptions in the specialty the applicant has selected.

Signature ______________________

Name ______________________
(please print)
Authority: ☐ Current CDT ☐ Licensed Dentist

Mailing address ______________________

____

Telephone ______________________

Fax ______________________

E-mail ______________________

Signature ______________________

Name ______________________
(please print)
Authority: ☐ Current CDT ☐ Licensed Dentist

Mailing Address ______________________

____

Telephone ______________________

Fax ______________________

E-mail ______________________

IX. EMPLOYER'S AFFIDAVIT

The NBC requires that a present or former employer sign this application. The NBC will view the signature of such employer as evidence of that individual's opinion that you are qualified to sit for certification examinations and that the information presented in this document is consistent with the employer's information.

To the attesting persons: Your signature below testifies that you are familiar with the skills and abilities of this CDT applicant, and that you are satisfied with the applicant's competence to fill dental prescriptions in the specialty the applicant has selected. It also indicates that the information contained in this application is consistent with your information regarding the applicant.

Signature ______________________ Date ______________________

Name ______________________ ☐ Present Employer ☐ Former Employer
(please print)

Mailing Address ______________________

____

Telephone ______________________ Fax ______________________

E-mail ______________________

continued...

All Certified Dental Technician Examinations Application, continued.

X. APPLICANT'S AFFIDAVIT

To the National Board for Certification in Dental Laboratory Technology (NBC):

I have read and understand the application instructions and the CDT Examination Handbook and I agree to submit to examinations as prescribed by the NBC.

I agree to indemnify and hold harmless the NBC, its Trustees, officers, employees and agents, and the institution where the CDT examination is administered from any and all liability for injury or damages suffered by me, or which I might cause to others, during the course of taking my examination.

I agree to submit to testing for certification according to the requirements and procedures specified by the NBC.

I further agree to abide by the laws and regulations which govern the practice of dentistry and the providing of dental laboratory technology services, restorations and devices to the dental profession.

I affirm that all statements made by me in this application are true and correct to the best of my knowledge. I understand that any misrepresentation of fact made in this application for testing or in future applications to the NBC for certification testing or renewal, or in my personal claim to certification (use of the CDT designation and logo), may be found cause for suspension or denial of certification or eligibility for certification testing.

I hereby verify that I have _____ years of education and/or employment in dental laboratory technology.

Applicant's Signature ______________________________ Date ______________

XI. PAYMENT

All CDT Exams Fee ☐ $835

Any applications submitted after the published deadline must be accompanied by a late fee of $100 ($25 per written exam and $50 for the Practical exam) and are subject to NBC approval.

☐ Enclosed is Check #__________ in the amount of $____________________ payable to the NBC.

☐ Please charge my credit card ☐ VISA ☐ MC ☐ AMEX Amount $________________

Credit Card #______________________________ Exp. ____________ CCV Code* __________

* Credit Card Verification (CCV Code): This is the 3-digit number that appears on the reverse side of your credit card. For American Express cards only, this is the 4-digit number on the front of your card.

Cardholder Name ______________________________ Signature ______________________

Billing Address ____

Phone ____

The fees published in this application are subject to change. Please verify fees with the NBC Headquarters before submitting this application. Write, call or visit the web site of the National Board for Certification in Dental Laboratory Technology at www.nbccert.org. The web site contains updated examination fees, schedules and complete candidate information as well as information about other programs.

If you have not signed your application or enclosed the required fees, your application will not be processed.

Please send completed application and fee to:
NBC
325 John Knox Road, #L103
Tallahassee, FL 32303
(850) 222-0053 Fax

Written Exam

1. Identify the following direct retainers
   a. Stress equalizers
   b. Minor connectors
   c. Precision attachment
   d. I-bars

2. The function of the reciprocal clasp arm is to
   a. Act as a direct retainer
   b. Perform as an indirect retainer
   c. Counteract any force transmitted by the retentive arm
   d. Stabilize the abutment teeth

3. Which of the following is a support element?
   a. Retentive mesh
   b. Clasp
   c. Occlusal rest
   d. Lingual bar

4. The purpose of beading along the border of palatal bar is to
   a. Stimulate tissue
   b. Prevent denture movement
   c. Keep food from getting between the bar and the base
   d. Prevent food from getting under the bar

5. Lingual plates and kennedy bars are
   a. Saddle retentions
   b. Major connectors
   c. Indirect retainers
   d. Tissue stops

6. An imaginary line drawn through the abutment teeth around which a partial would tend to rotate is called a
   a. Survey line
   b. Fulcrum line
   c. Line of demarcation
   d. Transverse

7. Compared to a gold alloy framework a chrome-cobalt alloy framework is

a. Easier to adjust
b. Thinner
c. More flexible
d. Easier to repair

8. A circumferential clasp approaches an undercut from the

a. Distal surface of the tooth
b. Mesial surface of the tooth
c. Gingival portion of the tooth
d. Occlusal portion of the tooth

9. Thermal expasion of a casting investment is accomplished

a. In a water bath
b. In the furnace
c. During setting time
d. During spatulation

10. A clasp must encircle the tooth at least degrees to prevent tooth movement

a. 90 degrees
b. 130 degrees
c. 180 degrees
d. 390 degrees

11. Correct wire size for fabricating a stainless steel wire molar clasp is

a. 0.016
b. 0.020
c. 0.036
d. 0.066

12. The tooth numbering system used today that is most common is

a. International
b. Palmer
c. Military
d. London

13. Type Ⅲ alloys are used for

a. Ceramic metal substructure
b. R.P.D. frameworks
c. Inlays
d. Three unit full metal bridges

14. Two adjacent teeth touch at the

a. Interproximal contact　　b. Occlusal

c. Cusp tips　　d. Marginal ridge

15. The distal surface of #29 will contact the

a. Mesial of #28　b. Distal of # 28　c. Distal of #30　d. Mesial of #30

16. The maximum contact attainable between maxillary and mandibilar teeth describes

a. Protrusive contacts　　b. Centric relation

c. Centric occlusion　　d. Balancing occlusion

17. Warm flasks are removed from the curing unit they should be allowed to cool in an effort to avoid

a. Porosity　b. Warpage　c. Contraction　d. Expansion

18. The numbers of casting machine turns for a base metal or non precious alloy will be

a. Decreased　　b. Increased

c. Same as precious alloy　　d. b and c

19. Dental porcelain's chief advantage is

a. Shade variation　b. Hardness　c. Strength　d. Esthetics

20. A bubble appears in the porcelain which extends to the metal this is caused by

a. Thermal shock　b. Too much opaque　c. Metal contamination　d. Over firing

(출처 : http://cafe.daum.net/usadentec)

Denturist

미국, 캐나다(denturist), 영국(clinical dental technician), 호주(dental prosthetist)에서 국소의치나 총의치의 제작과 수리 및 환자에게 직접적으로 수술을 포함하지 않는 시술을 할 수 있도록 교육을 받고 자격을 갖춘 사람을 의미한다.

Education and licensing

2~3년의 의치사가 되기 위한 교육 프로그램을 이수하고 완벽한 시술을 위해 실습 과정을 거친 후 각 주나 시에서 정한(주, 시에 따라 자격조건이 다름) 면허증을 획득하여야 한다.

Duties

- 환자의 구강 문제를 해결하기 위한 정보 수집
- 환자의 구강 내·외 검사
- 인상채득과 모형 제작
- 임시의치 제작
- 보철물의 구강 내 장착과 시적
- 직원 채용(치과위생사, 상담사 등)

1860년대 치과산업의 급격한 성장으로 인해 치과계에 다양한 전문 분야가 생겨났다. 그 결과 가철성 의치 제작 분야에 Denturism이 새롭게 만들어졌으며, 의치사들은 경험을 통해 지식을 습득하였다. 지금 현재 캐나다에는 4개의 대학교에서 의치사를 위한 과정을 개설하고 있다.

의치사 과정의 학생들은 최소한 3년의 교육과정을 수료해야 하며 환자 진료와 가철성 보철물 제작도 습득해야 한다. 구강 내 진료와 기공 과정을 이론과 실습을 통해 배워야 한다.

의치사는 독립적으로 개업을 할 수 있다. Denturism은 1961년 합법적으로 승인을 받은 후 많은 발전을 해왔다.

※ 의치사를 위한 웹사이트(http://www.international-denturists.org) 참조

General requirements for admission to school programs

- 고등학교 졸업자 이상 지원 가능
- 전문대 졸업자나 최소 2년의 자연과학 전공자 지원 가능

Colleges of Denturism

Program contents

• General Anatomy and Physiology	• Preventive Dentistry
• Orofacial Anatomy	• General Histology
• Dental Histology and Embryology	• Partial Dentures
• Microbiology	• Radiographic Interpretation
• Oral Pathology and Medicine	• Pre-clinical Prosthetics
• Psychology in Dentistry	• Clinical Prosthetics
• Dental Psychology and the Aging Patient	• Dentures Over Implants
• Complete Denture Prosthodontics	• Dental Materials
• Small Business Management	• Practice Management
• Pharmacology and Emergency Care	• Human Relations
• Dental Kinesiology	• Public Health, Legislation and Research
• Removable Partial Dentures	

memo

Chapter 4

Phone Call

1. 전화 걸고 받기

Key expressions

1. Make a call

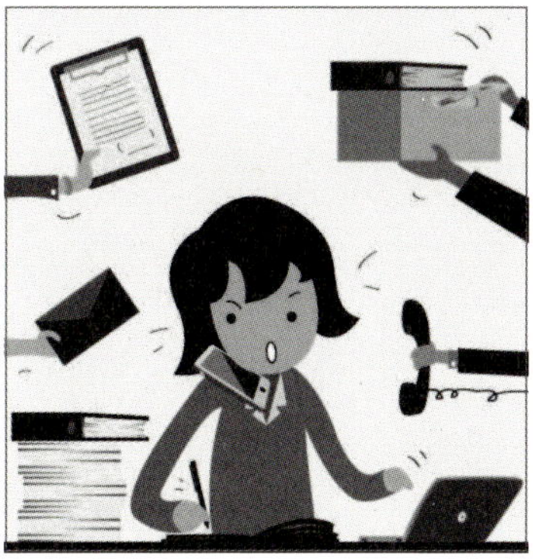

A : Hello. Is this Mr. Kim?

B : No, this is Ms. Lee, a secretary.

A : Oh, This is Myoung-su from Muhan. I called about payment. May I speak to Mr. Kim?

B : He is not in here now.

A : When will he be back?

B : Maybe after lunch.

A : OK. I will call back later. / Would you just tell him that I called, please?

B : OK. Anything else?

A : No, thank you. Bye.

2. Answer the phone

(Ringing)

A : Hello. This is Jun-ha in design department speaking.

B : Hello. This is Haha from Muhan. Can I talk to Mr. Kim?

A : What are you calling about?

B : I want to change meeting hour.

A : Oh, I see. Hold on please. Let me transfer your call. Oh, but he is on another line.

B : Then, Can I leave a message?

A : Of course.

Vocabulary

** You should say "this is", you refer to yourself when answer or talk with the phone.

- **Hold on** : Hold the phone line open
- **Transfer** : Be connected; I'll put you through

2. 팩스 보내기

[Street Address]
[City, ST Zip Code]
[phone]
[fax]
[Web address]

[Company Name]

Fax

To:	**From:**
Fax:	**Pages:**
Phone:	**Date:**
Re:	**cc:**

☐ **Urgent** ☐ **For Review** ☐ **Please Comment** ☐ **Please Reply** ☐ **Please Recycle**

● **Comments:** Select this text and delete it or replace it with your own. To save changes to this template for future use, choose Save As from the File menu. In the Save As Type box, choose Document Template. Next time you want to use it, choose New from the File menu, and then double-click your template.

3. Delivery

Dialogue : Call from dental clinic

A : EZ Dental lab. How may I help you?

B : Good morning! I am calling from Jang's Dental Clinic. We have a pickup today.

A : Okay. And also I have a delivery to your clinic.
The name of the patient is EunKyung Park.
Six unit zirconia bridges. When is the best time?

B : The patient will arrive at 2 pm, so before lunch time would be great.

A : All right. And, I will send the teeth pictures of the patient by email.
It is 4 anterior teeth from 7 to 10 and a very hard case.
Please check before you start the case.
And the patient must leave for Japan next Friday.
So, can you make it extra quickly?

B : I am really busy, but I will try.
And you know that there is en extra rush charge. It is $50.

A : No problem. Thank you. By the way, the patient is very sensitive.
If you have free time before you start, can the patient visit your lab?

B : Let me check my schedule first. Before noon on Friday could be great.
How about the patient?

A : Let me ask her. At 11 o'clock. Is it okay?

B : Great. The patient has to pay an extra shade taking charge. It is $30.

A : All right.

Sample prescription

Kim's Dental Care

Patient : ____________________

□ Digital Dental Lab;
386 Sejong-Ro,
Dong-Gu, Seoul.
02-887-2804

□ Fine Dental Lab;
27-5 Seo-Ro,
Buk-Gu, Daegu.
053-320-2804

□ Elite Dental Lab;
245 Kangbuk-Ro,
Kyeyang-Gu, Incheon.
032-287-2804

□ Name :
Address :
Phone :

Doctor : ____________________
Address : ____________________
____
Phone : ____________________
Fax : ____________________

Date of Rx: ____________________
Return Date : ____________________
Patient Appt : ____________________
Shade : ____________________
Tissue or Prep shade : ____________________

TEETH NUMBERS

1	2	3	4	5	6	7	8	9	10	11	12	13	14	15	16
32	31	30	29	28	27	26	25	24	23	22	21	20	19	18	17

Porcelain Fused to Metal	All Metals	All Ceramic
□ Porcelain to Non-Precious	□ Non-Precious(White)	□ e.max
□ Porcelain to Semi Precious	□ Non-Precious(Yellow)	□ PG Pro e.max(ADL)
□ Porcelain to White High Noble	□ Semi-Precious(White)	□ PG Pro BruxZir*(ADL)
□ Porcelain to Yellow High Noble	□ Yellow Gold	□ Porcelain to Zirconia
□ Maryland Bridge	□ Post & Core Non-Precious	□ Full Zirconia - BruxZir*(ADL)
□ Captek	□ Post & Core Semi-Precious	□ Full Zirconia - NexxZir (IDA)
	□ Post & Core Yellow Gold	

Margin Design

□ Porcelain Butt Margin
□ Lingual Collar in Metal
□ Full Metal Band
□ Full Metal Lingual □% □%
□ No Metal Collar

Partials and Dentures

□ Valplast
□ Acrylic
□ Premium Denture
□ Cast Framework
□ Base Plate/Bite Rim
□ Custom Tray
□ Try-In
□ Complete
□ Occlusal Guard
○ Upper or Lower
○ Hard/Hard
○ Hard/Soft

Dr's Signature____________ License #__________

THE STYLE

DENTAL LABORATORY

□ Phone : 02-9745-3804
□ Fax : 02-9764-5200
□ Address : Suite 309, Level 3, strathfield Plaza
11 The Boulevarde Strathfield NSW 2135
□ Emial : thestyledental@gmai.com

CLINIC

SHADE

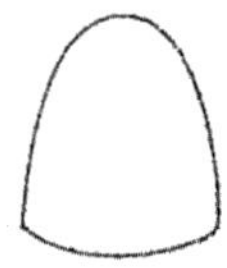

DENTIST

PATIENT NAME

DATE OF BIRTH M / F

SENT DATE

DUE DATE

INSTRUCTION

** If no selection is made we will carry out the job with normal settings.

1. Job Type :
   - ☐ VMK ☐ E-Max press ☐ Zirconia
   - ☐ Gold Crown ☐ Gold Inlay ☐ Ceramic Inlay ☐ Laminate

2. Metal :
   - ☐ Precious ☐ Semi-precious ☐ Non-precious

3. Margin Design :
   - ☐ 360° Porcelain Margin ☐ Buccal Porcelain Margin
   - ☐ No-Metal ☐ Lingual Metal

4. Implant :
   - ☐ Cement ☐ Screw ☐ SCRP

Kim's Dental Studio

Suite 309, Level 3, strathfield Plaza
11 The Boulevarde Strathfield NSW 2135
Phone: 02-9745-3804 Fax : 02-9764-5200

TEETH NUMBERS															
1	2	3	4	5	6	7	8	9	10	11	12	13	14	15	16
32	31	30	29	28	27	26	25	24	23	22	21	20	19	18	17

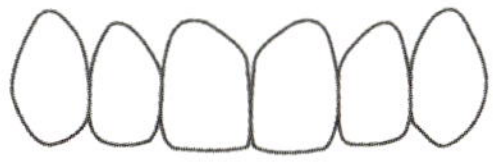

Shade of preps (stump) ______

Final Shade ______

Dr. Name ______ Pt. Name ______

Address ______ Sex ______ Age ______

______

Phone ______

NOTE: If no due date is assigned, a standard due date will be applied. Please call to schedule combination cases.

Dentist License # ______

Rx date

Dr. Signature (required)

Due date

______

Person signing this authorization accepts sole responsibility for payment and agrees to pay all legal fees.

Surface texture	Incisal translucency	Occlusal stain	In casse of inadequate clearence:
□ Smooth	□ Minimum (0.5mm)	□ None	□ Spot opposing
□ Moderate	□ Moderate (1mm)	□ Light	□ Reduction coping
□ Heavy	□ Heavy (1.5mm)	□ Medium	□ Metal stop
		□ Dark	□ Call me.

RESTORATIONS

All Ceramic
- □ Emax
- □ Zr.XT(100% Xr. 600MPa)
- □ Zr, (100% Zr. 1200 MPa)
- □ Empress Esthetic
- □ Porcelain fused to Zr.

Composit
- □ Tescera / Boscp

Full Gold / Metal
- □ Gold -75% AU
- □ WHT. Metal -40% AU, 40% PD

Porcelain Fused to Metal
- □ High Noble white
- □ Noble white

Metal Design
- □ Porcelain Butt
- □ 360 metal margin (0.5mm)
- □ Lingual band only

Removable
- □ Frame + bite block
- □ Denture teeth set-up
- □ Denture finish
- □ Wax Rim

Implant Type ______

Cement Retained (choose one)

Abutment	Crown
□ Zir.	□ Zirkon
□ Ti	□ Emax
□ Gold	□ PFM

Screw Retained
- □ Zirkon w/Ti insert
- □ Emax w/Ti insert

Orthosis
- □ Removable
- □ Fixed LVI

ALL on 4
- □ Screw Retained w/Ti bar
- □ Screw Retained Zir.
- □ Hybrid Bar over Denture *Dr.specifys type
- □ Surgical Stent

DIAGNOSTIC WAX-UP AND COMPREHENSIVE CASES (Must for Anterior Cases)

Photos for Wax-up
- □ Facial with smile
- □ Smile with lip
- □ Dental close-up (retracted)
- □ Profile smile

Photos for Final
- □ Prep shade
- □ Facial with smile in temps
- □ Smile with lip
- □ Dental close-up (retracted)
- □ Profile smile

For Mounting, please send us:
- □ Symmetry bite
- □ Kois Occl. Anal.
- □ Facebow transfer
- □ Fox plane
- □ Other

Smile Design
- □ L.V.I. Smile Catalog ____
- □ Smile Guide by Dorfman ____
- □ Match Photos
- □ Follow temps mockup
- □ Other ____

Length of Centrals

Original: #8 ____
#9 ____
Final: #8 ____
#9 ____

- □ Width buccal corridor teeth #______ ______mm
- □ Tissue re-contouring teeth #______ ______mm

Send back to Dr. w/D-wax-up
- □ Temp stent
- □ Incisal reduction stent
- □ Facial reduction stent
- □ Prep model.

SPECIAL INSTRUCTION

Have you included the following:
- □ Impressions
- □ Bite registration
- □ Pre-op model
- □ Opposing
- □ Photos
- □ Symmetry/Facebow

Please send:
- □ Rx's
- □ Boxes
- □ Airbills

For lab use:

Kim's Dental Lab

Suite 309, Level 3, strathfield Plaza
11 The Boulevarde Strathfield NSW 2135

Phone: 02-9745-3804
Fax : 02-9764-5200

Date Sent	
Return Date	
Patient Appt	

Doctor : ______________________

Patient : ______________________

Tooth No : ______________________

Shade : ______________________

Sex : ________ Age : __________

SPECIFIC INSTRUCTIONS

ITEMS ENCLOSED

Impression
- □ Upper
- □ Lower
- □ Triple Tray
- □ Opposing
- □ Bite
- □ Pick up Impression
- □ Partial
- □ Old Crown/Bridge

CROWN AND BRIDGE

Metal
- □ Non Precious
- □ Semi Precious
- □ White High Noble
- □ Yellow High Noble
- □ Full Gold
- □ Goldtek (Bio 2000)

All Ceramic
- □ Full Zirconia
- □ Zirconia
- □ Emax
- □ Veneer

Margin Design
- □ Porcelain Butt Margin-Facial
- □ Metal Margin ________ mm
- □ Show no Metal
- □ Metal Lingual Collar

Process
- □ Coping Try-in
- □ Bisque Bake Try-in
- □ Finish

When Occlusion is Tight :

- □ Spot Opposing
- □ Metal Island
- □ Spot Prep
- □ Call Doctor
- □ Reduction Coping

DESIGN CASE

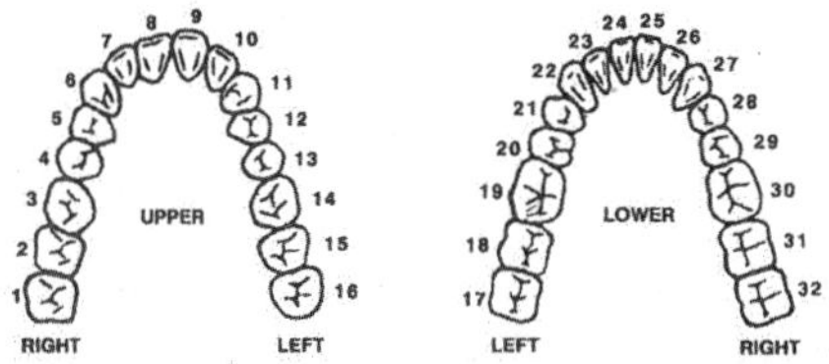

REMOVABLE RESTORATIONS

- □ Full Upper
- □ Full Lower
- □ Partial Upper
- □ Partial Lower
- □ Immediates
- □ Flipper
- □ Valplast

MISCELLANEOUS

- □ Custom Tray
- □ Night Guard
- □ Attachment
- □ Reline
- □ Teeth Repair
- □ Acrylic Repair
- □ Clasp Repair

DENTURE PROCESS

- □ Resin-Base & Wax Rim
- □ Metal Frame & Wax Rim
- □ Teeth Arrangement
- □ Cure and Finish

Dr's Signature ______________________ License #__________

THE STYLE DENTAL CERAMICS

Chart for Comparing Restorative Alternative 2015

	CORE SUPPORTED PORCELAIN RESTORATION			MONOLITHIC ZIRCONIA	MONOLITHIC LiSi2
	PFM	PFZ (Coping)	PFZ with ZR Occlusion!	FZ	e.g. 'e.Max'
Minimum Labial Reduction	1.5 mm	1.5 mm	1.5 mm	1.0 mm	0.7 mm
Margin Preparation Design	Facial Heavy Shoulder Facial Heavy Chamfer	Heavy Chamfer	Heavy Chamfer	Heavy Chamfer	Chamfer
Capacity to have Porcelain Butt Margin	Yes	No	No	No	N/A
Resistance to Chipping	Fair~100 mp	Fair~100 mp	Excellent~800 MP	Excellent~800 MP	Good~400 MP
Resistance to Fracture	Excellent! Core=1500 MP	Excellent! Core=1000 MP	Excellent-800 MP	Excellent~800 MP	Fair-400 MP
Core Thickness	Min. 0.5 mm	Min. 0.7 mm	Min. 0.7 mm	Monolithic: No Core	Monolithic: No Core
Translucency	Must be "Developed". It is an ILLUSION!	Must be "Developed". It is an ILLUSION!	It is an ILLUSION! More opaque than PFZ Coping!	Opacious!	Naturally Excellent!
Blocking Light?	100%	50~60%	60~80%	80~90%	10~20%
Repairability	Indirect : Porcelain	Indirect : Porcelain	Indirect : Porcelain	Indirect : Porcelain	Indirect : Porcelain
Posterior Inlay/Onlay	No	No	No	Yes (With Reservation)	Yes
Anterior Full Crown	Yes	Yes	Yes	No	Yes
Veneer	No	No	No	No	Yes
Bicuspid Full Crown	Yes	Yes	Yes	Yes (With Reservation)	Yes
Molar Full Crown	Yes (Metal Occl. Rec.)	No	No	Yes	No
Anterior Bridge	Yes	Yes	Yes	No	Yes (With Reservations)
Posterior Bridge	Yes	No	Yes	Yes	No
Cementation Requirements	Dentist's Chice	Dentist's Chice (No Etching!)	Dentist's Chice (No Etching!)	Dentist's Chice (No Etching!)	Best with Full Resin Bonding
Relative Surface Abrasiveness	Slightly More Than Natural Enamel	Slightly More Than Natural Enamel	Like Natural Enamel	Like Natural Enamel	Slightly More Than Natural Enamel

Suite 309, Level 3, strathfield Plaza 11 The Boulevarde Strathfield NSW 2135
Phone : 02-9745-3804 Fax : 02-9764-5200

THE STYLE DENTAL CERAMICS Ltd

Crown & Bridge

THE STYLE DENTAL CERAMICS Ltd

Suite 309, Level 3, strathfield Plaza 11
The Boulevarde Strathfield NSW 2135
Tel : 02-9745-3804 Fax : 02-9764-5200

In office use only :

M: ____________________	C: ____________________
Mt: __________ Wt: __________	In: __________ Cer: __________

DATE: ____________________ DR's PHONE: (______) ______________

Dr. ____

PATIENT NAME: ____

☐ MALE ☐ FEMALE

RETURN DATE: ____________________ RETURN TIME: __________AM/PM

Rx: ____

____

____

____

____

____

____

____

☐ **Custom Shade - In Lab** (for appt please call)

Final Tooth Shade(s): ____________________ Stump Shade: ______________

DOCTOR'S SIGNATURE: ____

Please indicate case requirements below:

Centric Contact:	☐ Positive	☐ Shim Relief	☐ Double Relief
Pontic Design:	☐ Hygienic	☐ Ridge Lap	☐ Ovate _____mm
Lat. Excursion:	☐ Cuspid Guidance	☐ Group Function	☐ Cross Bite
Occlusion:	☐ Ceramic	☐ Metal in Centric	☐ All Metal
Facial Margin:	☐ Ceramic Butt	☐ Combination	☐ Fine Metal
PFM Metal:	☐ High AU (70~90%)	☐ Mid Au (40~60%)	☐ Semi-Precious
	☐ Yellow Semi-Precious (FGC only)		☐ CrCo (Non-Prec)

Core Supporrted All-Ceramics:

Zirconia:	☐ Porcelain Fused to Zirconia (PFZ)		☐ Full Contour (FZ)
Lithium DiSilicate:	☐ e-Max	☐ Other ______________	

Core Free All-Ceramics:

Feldspathic:	☐ Prep	☐ No-Prep	☐ Other __________
Pressed:	☐ Empress	☐ e-Max	☐ Other __________

Lingual/Occlusal Metal Design:

 ☐ Metal Lingual Collar

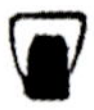 ☐ 3/4 Metal Lingual

 ☐ Full Metal Lingual

 ☐ High Lingual Collar

 ☐ Metal Lingual Collar

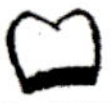 ☐ Metal Margin

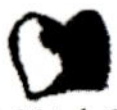 ☐ 1/2 Metal Occlusal

 ☐ Full Metal Occlusal

 ☐ Metal Island

4. Instructions

Sample #1

Please fabricate All-Ceramic Zirconia 12

Crown in shade A3. I have emailed the photograph of the original tooth before prep. thank you.

Sample #2

Please fabricate PFM crown 11, buccal porcelain & lingual metal.

I will send picture of 11 for crown fabrication via email titled under the patient's name for reference of esthetics.

Sample #3

Metal occlusal surface, light occlusal contact (0.5mm). Patient is heavy biter.

Buccal porcelain margin, lingual metal margin.

Shade A3.5 for porcelain, normal interproximal contact.

Sample #4

Nickel free None-precious metal. A3 color

Sample #5

pls, tight interproximal contacts, minimal occlusal contacts

Excellent margin fit. If any problem, call me before

Sample #6

46 PFM crown

360° porcelain margin, light occlussion, good contacts very important!!

Sample #7

Attention : (Esthetic case) All zirconia

6 unit bridge with original pink porcelain to cover the back of soft tissue.

Patient is a Doctor and very ware about esthetic of her front teeth.

She has a high smile line and wants her centrals length to almost 11mm long. Make sure the laterals are symmetrical in the shape.

PS. She is kinda happy with her temporary, I took alginate impression of her temporary. Please make them to look very natural.

Sample #8

Case Description

Qty	Product Description	Tooth#'s
8	Emax Crown/Veneer(Asthetic Case 6+)	6,7,8,9,10,11,12,13
2	Emax Inlay	4,5

Shade : BL1-Brightest shade

Veneer # 4-13(#3+5 are emax onlays)

#1 Two impressions included

- Impression labeled #1 : tooth #5 has facial void
- Impression labeled #2 : tooth #5 looks good, but #8 was reprepped(It is correct)

#2 Patient wants laterals slightly(0.5mm) on impression #1 - shorter and tapered (more feminine)

7/29 - Wrote a return note- and Returned the entire case back to Dr.Kim to be prepped more

7/31 received the case back.(has been prepped more)

Sample #9

Attn : Jenny

- Plan is for Full Zirconia bridge
- Do not make embrasure too tight.
- Jenny. Please look at this case and let me know if you think that would be problematic. We can do PFM if necessary. Please call me.

memo

Chapter 5

Post Office

1. 우체국

Key expressions

■ At post office

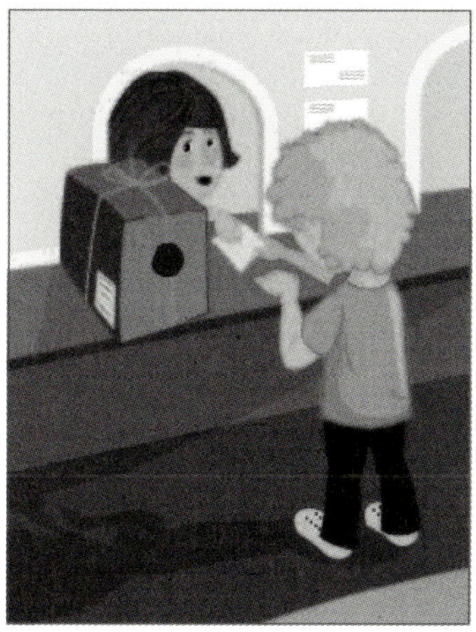

A : I'd like an envelope, please.

B : OK. Here it is.

A : Where is the postbox?

B : The postbox is in front of the door.

A : I'd like to send this letter to Korea.

B : OK. Can you fill in this form please?

A : Yeah. Here you are. I'd like to send this letter by recorded delivery. How much will it cost to send this?

B : 12.50 dollars, please.

A : I'd like to send this parcel to Brazil.

B : OK. Can you put it on the scale, please?

A : I've come to collect a parcel.

B : Oh, here it is.

Vocabulary

- **Envelope** : A flat (usually rectangular) container for a letter, thin package, etc
- **Postbox** : Public box for deposit of mail
- **Recorded delivery** : Providing permanent evidence of delivery
- **Parcel** : A wrapped container
- **Scale** : A measuring instrument for weighing; shows amount of mass

2. 분실 기공물 찾기

Dialogue : Finding lost property

A : Good afternoon, Digital Dental Lab. How may I help you?

B : Hi. I'm calling from Kim's Clinic.

I have not received the prosthesis which should have arrived this morning.

A : What is the patient's name?

B : Jenny Choi. 4 units zirconia bridge.

A : I already sent that case last Tuesday.

B : What's the name of delivery company?

A : FEDEX.

B : Let me have the tracking number please.

A : Okay. It's 792337037540

B : Let me check.

Oh. It's here. Someone took it, and left it in the wrong place. Anyway, thanks.

3. 택배회사

Get rates & Transit times

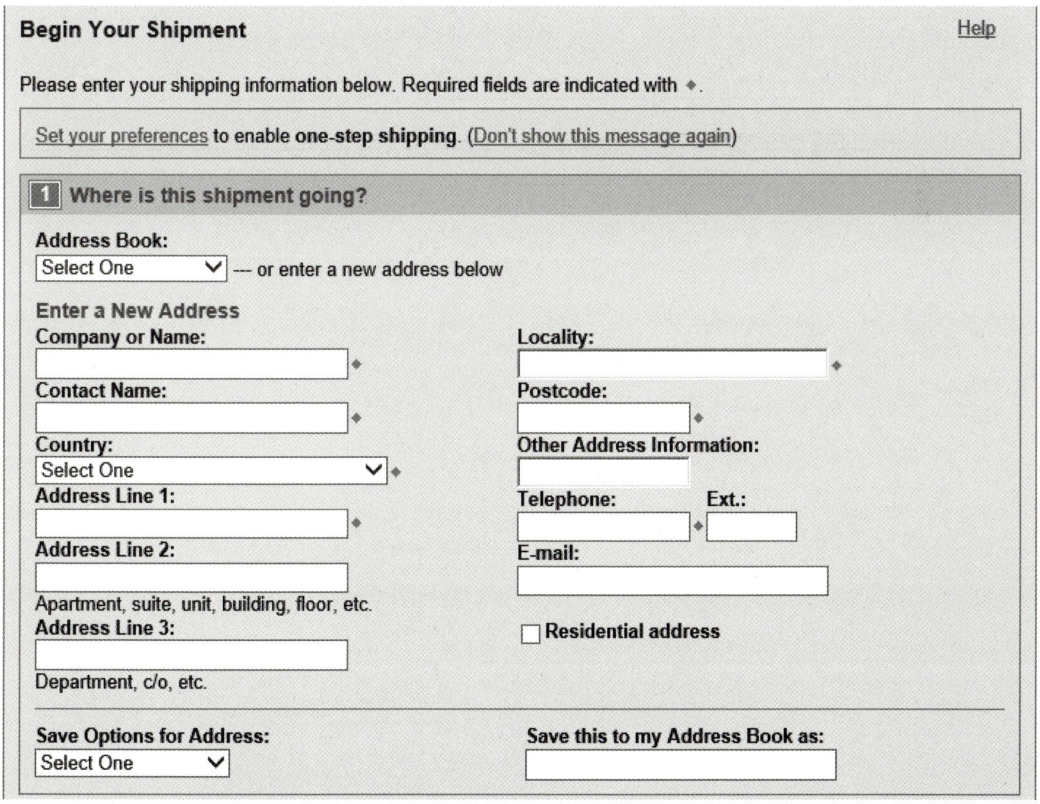
Begin Your Shipment Help

Please enter your shipping information below. Required fields are indicated with ◆.

Set your preferences to enable **one-step shipping**. (Don't show this message again)

1 Where is this shipment going?

Address Book:
Select One --- or enter a new address below

Enter a New Address

Company or Name: ◆
Contact Name: ◆
Country: Select One ◆
Address Line 1: ◆
Address Line 2:
Apartment, suite, unit, building, floor, etc.
Address Line 3:
Department, c/o, etc.

Locality: ◆
Postcode: ◆
Other Address Information:
Telephone: ◆ **Ext.:**
E-mail:
☐ **Residential address**

Save Options for Address:
Select One

Save this to my Address Book as:

2 Where is this shipment coming from?

Ship From Address: Edit
se hyun lee
se hyun lee
Deagu
Deagu 30111
South Korea
Telephone:+820 3950 9357

If the shipment is undeliverable return to :

Contact:
se hyun lee

Return Address:
Same As Ship From

3 What are you shipping?

Description of Goods:

☐ Documents of No Commercial Value

Number of Packages:
1

Packages are all the same?
Yes

Packaging Type:
Select One

4 How would you like to ship?

Service:
Select Service

Compare Time and Cost

Do you need additional services?	**Fee?**
☐ Send E-mail Notifications	Free
☐ Receive Confirmation of Delivery	Yes
☐ Deliver On Saturday	Yes
☐ Direct Delivery Only	Yes
☐ Offset the climate impact of this shipment (UPS carbon neutral)	Yes

Some services may require extra information. You will be able to enter the required information on the next page.

5 Would you like to add reference numbers to this shipment?

UPS gives you the option to track your shipments using references that you define.

Reference#1

[ ]

Reference#2

[ ]

☐ Add a bar code for Reference#1 to my Shipping label

6 How would you like to pay?

Please enter your payment information below. The information you enter will be transmitted using a secure connection. Required fields are indicated with ◆.

Bill Shipping Charges to:

Select One ◆

Promotion Code:

[ ] Apply Code

Bill Duties and Taxes to:

Select One ◆

☐ Split Duty / VAT

7 Would you like to schedule a collection?

☐ Schedule a UPS On-Call Collection.

☑ Review Shipping details, including price, before completing this shipment

Start Over | Next »

Track the way you want

- Need the status of your shipment or a proof of delivery?
- Enter your tracking number or reference number below.

Track it now

- **Tracking number**
- Track by Reference
- Obtain Proof of Delivery

Help

Enter up to 30 FedEx tracking numbers (one per line).

Enter up to 30

Track

Tracking number	792337037540	**Destination**	SEOCHO GU SEOUL KR
Ship date	Jul 20, 2005		
Estimated delivery	Jul 27, 2005 6:00 PM	**Service type**	Priority Envelope
		Weight	0.5 kgs.
Status	Package data transmitted to FedEx		

Date/Time	Activity	Location	Details
Jul 20, 2005 3:57 PM	**Package data transmitted to FedEx**		

Chapter 6

Housing

1. 집 구하기 (Rent)

Key expressions

1. At property (Real estate)

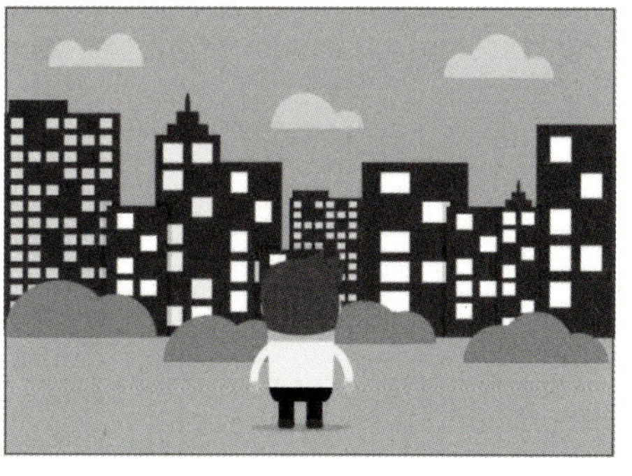

A : May I help you?

B : I am looking for a one-bedroom apartment.

A : What price range are you looking at?

B : About 500 dollars a month.

A : Hi. I am calling about the apartment for rent. Is it still available?

B : Yes, it is.

A : I would like to see it. Would you mind if I ask a few questions about the studio first?

B : Yes, please. What do you want to know?

A : What is included in the rent?

B : The rent includes utilities.

A : How much is the security deposit?

B : 1,000 dollars, a month rent fee.

A : How long is the lease?

B : One year.

A : Is a short-term lease available?

B : I have to check with landlord about that.

A : Can I move in now?

B : No, you can move in after July 17.

2. Repair

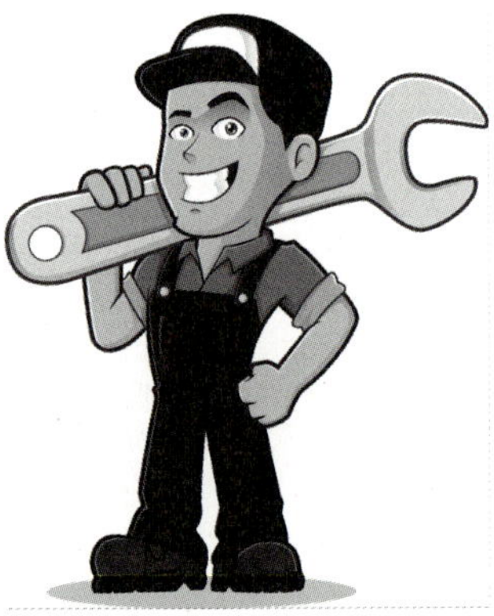

A : The microwave is broken.

The air conditioner isn't cold enough.

The refrigerator doesn't work.

The sink is clogged.

The toilet won't flush.

The heat is out.

There is no hot water.

Vocabulary

- **Property (Real estate)** : Houses and land
- **Studio** : An apartment with a living space and a bathroom and a small kitchen
- **Utility** : The service (electric power or water or transportation) provided by a public utility
- **Deposit** : A payment given as a guarantee
- **Lease** : Property that is rented out or let
- **Landlord** : A land owner or a house owner
- **Move in** : Move into a new house or office
- **Refrigerator** : Which can store food at low temperatures
- **Clogged** : Stopped up
- **Flush** : A sudden rapid flow (as of water)

House advertising

Vocabulary

- 5 appl
- Abstainer
- Adult building
- Amenity
- Apt
- Avail. immed
- Bach
- Bachelor apt
- Balc
- Bath
- Bedsit riin
- Bldg
- Bsmt
- Bsmt suite
- Close to TTC
- Cls to all amen
- D.D
- Den
- Evgs
- First and last monst
- Flat
- Fully equipped all appliances

- Fun, Unfun
- Furn : Furnished
- IMMED
- Incls. Utils.
- Junior one bedroom
- Lease
- Lrg
- Mo
- Newly reno
- N/P
- N/S
- One bedroom
- RM
- Self-contained
- Share bathroom/kitchen
- Studio
- Sublet
- Suite
- U/G prk
- Utl. inch(peid)
- WK
- Wkends
- WW carpeting

Apartment features

- Cable Ready
- Gas Range
- Hardwood Flooring
- New/Renovated Interior
- Some Paid Utilities

Community Features

- Emergency Maintenance
- Garage
- Laundry Facility
- Playground
- Public Transportation
- Pet Friendly

Special Features

- Pets
- Call for Policy Weight restriction : 25

Additional Features

- Close to PATH train
- Garden apartments
- Easy access bus stop to New York City
- Newly renovated
- Close to downtown, shopping and restaurants
- Beautiful hardwood flooring
- Easily accessible to all major NJ freeways
- On site parking
- Close to excellent schools
- Garages available
- Heat and hot water inlcuded
- Laundry facilities on premises
- On-site management
- 24-hour maintenance
- Pets welcome-Call for policy

Apartment Info

Brookdale Gardens is built on twenty acres in a park-like setting surrounded by trees and open spaces. Bloomfield's biggest advantages are it's closeness to excellent schools, Bloomfield College and Hoffman LaRoche parks, transportation in N.J. and twenty minutes to N.Y.C. and a short distance to Newark's new cultural center and airports. All prices include hot water and heat!

Lease Terms

Variable

2. Delay

Dialogue : Delay the delivery date

A : Good morning, Kim's Clinic. How may I help you?

B : Hi. This is Jenny from Digital Dental Lab.

I have a problem.

I have to send a 6 units PFM bridge tomorrow, but I failed that case. Could you move the appointment date?

A : Okay. What is the patient's name?

B : It is InHo Jang.

A : Let me check. Here is the patient's information.

The appointment date is June 15th. So, when is the best time for you?

B : June 23rd would be great. I have to start that case from the first step.

A : Do I have to take a new impression again?

B : No, I have a duplicate model which I took as soon as I got the case.

A : Great! Then, is there any other problem to fabricate PFM?

B : Can you ask the patient to change the material?

Due to the patient's lack of occlusal bite, there is not enough space for ceramic.

The total thickness of the crown will be 1 mm.

Can you prep the teeth more? Or I would recommend zirconia.

A : Zirconia?

Okay. I will discuss this with the patient.

B : Okay. I will await your answer.

A : All right. Talk to you later.

- 30 minute later -

B : Hi. This is JunHo.

I talked to the patient.

The patient doesn't want to preb more.

So, change to zirconia please.

A : Thanks. I will do it right away.

3. 치과 거래 규정 (가격, 제작 기간 등)

Company's price list & policy

Porcelain Fused to Metal

PFM (+ 〉 1.0g of weighted alloy)		Non-Precious	$84
		Noble (Semi)	$104
		White High Noble	$129
	esthetic Design	+6 Unit	$159

Non Metal Crowns

Emax Crown/Veneer		Anterior	$159
IPS e.max		Posterior	$139
	esthetic Design	+6 Unit	$159
Zirconia		Anterior	$159
		Posterior	$135
	esthetic Design	+6 Unit	$159
Full Zirconia		Posterior	$139
	esthetic Design	+6 Unit	$159

Full Metal Crown / Inlay	+ all weighted alloy	$79
Cast Post & Core		$74

Implants

Custom UCLA Abutment + any Crown		Parts included	$269
Titanium Custom Abutment + any Crown*		Parts included	$369
Zirconia Custom Abutment + any Crown*		Parts included	$419
Titanium Encode Abutment + any Crown		Parts included	$599
Implant Screw Retained	+ alloy		$229
Implant Screw Retained(Ceramic)			$299

Dentures

Complete Denture	Set Up & Finish	$339
Bite Rim/Base Plate		$33
Partial Denture	Frame	$199
	Set Up	$114
	Finish	$114
Valplast Partial Denture		$339
Denture Teeth (per set)		$14
Same Day Denture Repair		$149

Others

Diagnostics Wax Up	per unit		$34
Diagnostics Additive Wax Up	per unit		$14
Model Duplication	per arch		$14
Putty Matrix (for temporaries)	per arch		$34
Stent-Prep Guided (Putty)	per arch		$14
Stent-Clear Prep Guided	per arch		$34
Temps (Provisinoal)	per unit		$54
Orthosis	Fixed/Removable	per arch	$259
Flipper (1 tooth & 1 clasp included)			$152
Bleaching Tray			$69
Night Guard	Hard, Hard/Soft		$164
	Soft		$89

Essix Retainer		$69

* Note : Days not including pick-up & delivery day
** Times provided are minimum number of business days

Classification		Days
PFM		10
Ceramics		10
Implants		10
Diagnostics		Calculated / Unit
Complete Dentures (Set Up & Finish)		10
Partials	Framework	10
	Set Up	8
	Finish	8
Valplast Partial		5
Flipper / Bleaching Tray / Night Guard / Essix Retainer		5

Rush Charge		Price
Completion in	5 Days	$25
	4 Days	$50
	3 Days	$75
	2 Days	$100
	1 Days	$150

For other inquires or to schedule a pick-up,
Please feel free to contact us at + 82-53-2XX-XXXX
Email : XXXX@XXXX.net

Agreement

X ______________________________ Date : ______________

X ______________________________

Chapter 7

Restaurant

Key expressions

1. Booking

A : I'd like to make a reservation.
Do you have any free tables?

B : When for?

A : This evening at seven thirty.

B : For how many people?

A : A table for four please.

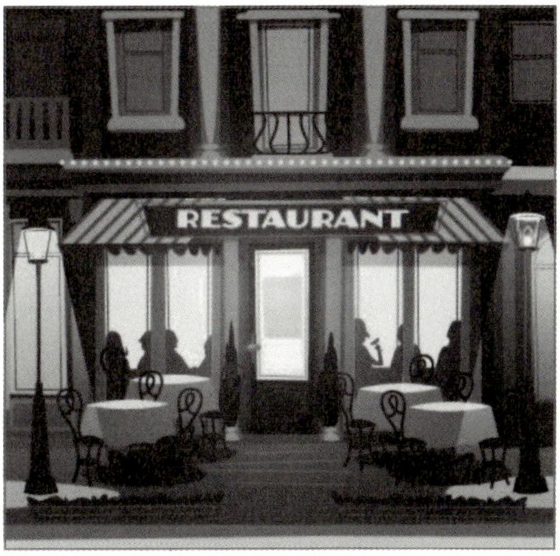

2. Ordering

A : Do you have a reservation?

B : Yes, I've got a reservation.

A : Could I see the menu please?

B : Yes, here it is.

A : (Point the menu) What is this dish?

B : Oh, This is a kind of pasta with cream sauce and variety of vegetables.

A : Oh! I'm severely allergic to dairy products. OK. wait a minute, please.

A : Are you ready to order?

B : I'll have the chicken salad, beef steak and two pastas.

A : I'm sorry, we're out of chicken salad.

B : Oh, then I'll take mushroom salad.

A : How would you like your steak?

B : Medium-rare, please.

A : OK. Would you like anything else?

B : Nothing else, thank you.

3. During the meal

(After serving)

B : Enjoy your meal!

A : Excuse me. Is our meal on its way?

B : Oh, OK. I'll check.

A : And Could we have some more bread?

B : OK. here you are.

A : Excuse me. This isn't what I ordered. And this is too salty.

B : Oh, I'm sorry I'll check it.

4. Paying

A : The bill, please.

B : Here you are.

DaehanNarae
Suite 309, Level 3, strathfield Plaza 11
The Boulevarde Strathfield NSW 2135
TEL : 02-9745-3804
www.DaehanNarae.com

CARD TYPE : MC
CARD HOLDER : XXXXXXXXXXXX
CARD NUMBER : XXXXXXXXXXXX
EXPIRATION DATE : XXXX

DATE : 2015-08-15 TIME : 1:57:34 PM

Invoice# : XXXXXXXX
Tabel# : B08
Server Name : Jenny Choi

Charge Amt $: 19.46
TIP AMOUNT $ ____________
FINAL AMT $ ____________

APPROVED : XXXXXX
TRACK # : XXXX

SIGNATURE : ____________________

-------------- THANK YOU --------------

Not itemized
Not reimbursable

DaehanNarae
Suite 309, Level 3, strathfield Plaza 11
The Boulevarde Strathfield NSW 2135
TEL : 02-9745-3804
www.DaehanNarae.com

Re-Pringting 1
Dine In
Date : 15-08-2015 Time : 1:57 PM # 30

Server : Jenny Choi
TAB : B08
No of Guest : 2

1 L-Cashew Chicken	7.50
w. Brown Rice	
w.Egg Flower Shop	
1 L-Mongolian Chicken	8.00
w. Brown Rice	
w.Egg Flower Shop	
1 Hot Tea (per pot)	2.50
Amount :	18.00
TAX(8.1%) :	1.46
TOTAL :	19.46

Thank you very much.

Itemized
Reimbursable

A : Is service included?

B : Oh, yes.

A : Can I pay by credit card?

B : Yes, of course. Was everything alright?

A : Yeah, delicious.

5. At fast food

A : Welcome to McDonald's. May I take your order?

B : I'll take a Big Mac and a small coke.

A : One Big Mac and one small coke. Will that be all?

B : Yes.

A : Here to go?

B : Here.

A : The total comes to $3.87.

Vocabulary

- **Booking** : The act of reserving
- **Reservation** : The act of reserving
- **Salty** : Filled with salt
- **Out of** : Sold out

Tip 문화

미국에서 팁이 필요한 곳은 식당, 술집, 택시, 미장원, 이발소, 호텔 등이다. 일반적으로 고객 개인에게 많은 시간과 노력을 베푸는 서비스에 팁을 주게 되어 있다. 식당의 경우 좌석에 앉아 주문을 하고 음식을 받는 경우가 그렇다. 따라서 고객이 카운터에서 주문을 하고 음식을 직접 받는 '테이크아웃' 식당이나 패스트푸드 체인 등은 팁을 주지 않아도 된다.

'점심 10% 저녁 15%' 또는 '점심 15% 저녁 20%'

식당에서 테이블 서비스를 받는 경우, 대개 음식 가격의 15~20%를 팁으로 준다. 미국 식당의 계산서를 보면 두 가지 금액이 찍혀 나오는 것을 볼 수 있다. 하나는 주문한 음식 가격이고, 다른 하나는 세금이다(세율은 지역에 따라 달라진다). 팁 계산은 세금을 제외한 음식가격만으로 한다. 택시 운전사, 미용사, 그리고 피자 등의 음식 배달원 역시 이 정도면 적당하다.

술집에서 주문하는 음료는 보통 1잔당 1달러로 계산한다. 바텐더에게서 음료를 직접 받아 오는 경우에도 팁을 남기는 것이 관례다. 만일 음료를 여러 잔 시키고, 음식도 함께 주문하는 경우는 전체 금액의 20%를 주면 된다. 뷔페식당에서는 (음식을 별도로 주문하지 않는 한) 1인당 1달러로 족하다.

호텔에서 짐을 날라 주는 포터의 경우 가방 하나당 1~2달러, 차를 대신 주차해 주는 사람(valet)에게는 2~5달러 정도를 준다. 호텔에서 룸서비스를 받는 경우 세금을 제외한 계산서 액수의 10~15%면 되지만, 청구금액에 서비스료가 포함되어 있는지 확인할 필요가 있다. 계산서만으로 잘 알 수 없을 경우 상대에게 물어도 큰 실례가 아니다. 식당이나 술집에서도 여러 명이 동석하는 경우는 계산서에 팁을 포함해 청구하기도 한다. 물론, 이 경우 별도로 팁을 주지 않는다.

팁 주기가 외국인들에게만 혼란스러운 것은 아니다. 미국인들 가운데 '점심 10%, 저녁 15%'를 고집하는 사람들도 있고, '점심 15%, 저녁 20%'는 되어야 한다고 말하는 이들도 있다. 하지만 어느 경우든 15% 정도를 주면 '고약한 팁 손님(bad tipper)'이라는 비난은 면할 수 있다. 물론, 서비스가 훌륭했다면 얼마든지 더 주어도 좋다.

[불만] "도대체 무슨 서비스를 한다고 팁을 줘?"

비록 팁 주는 비율이 높아지고 팁 서비스의 범위도 넓어졌지만, 미국에서 팁은 생략할 수 없는 고객의 의무다. 대다수 팁 노동자들에게 고객의 호의는 필수 불가결한 밥줄의 일부이기 때문이다. 미국의 공정노동법(FLAS)이 정한 2009년 연방최저임금은 시간당 7.25달러다. 그러나 2009년 6월 현재 미국의 식당종업원이 받는 시간당 평균임금은 4달러를 겨우 넘을 뿐이다.

Remake와 재료 추천

Dialogue 1 : Remake

A : Hi. Doctor Kim. How are you?

B : I'm good.

I have a remake case which is 4 units zirconia bridge.

The patient's name is EunSook Choi.

I tried it in the patient's mouth but the color is too dark.

A : Really? Let me find her record.

Here it is.

The shade is A2, and I matched to the Vita Shade Guide.

I think it was OK.

B : Yeah. But it's too dark and out of value.

A : Hum. Is it a vital tooth?

B : Yes, and it's a discolored tooth.

Sorry, I did't mention it on the prescription.

A : Oh. Then, zirconia is not the right choice because regular zirconia can't block the discolored tooth.

The best way is to change to PFM or use a bleach shade zirconia block for the discolored tooth.

B : A bleach shade zirconia block will be great because the patient has a metal allergy and does not like the black line at the margin of PFM.

A : All right. Change to bleach shade zirconia block.

Is there any request like shape or marginal fit?

B : Everything is great except the color.

A : Okay. And you know there is same charge in case of a remake?

B : I know that.

Could you send it by next Friday.

The patient is scheduled for her wedding on Sunday.

A : Okay. I will and the extra rush charge is her wedding gift.

B : I will tell her. Thank you.

Dialogue 2 : Materials and design recommendation

A : Good morning doctor Park.

B : Hi. Mr. Ahn. I need your help.

I have a partial denture case.

It is on the upper side and he is very sensitive which means major connector will make him gag.

Is there any other way without major connector?

A : Since it is a partial denture case, the design cannot be completed with a major connector.

How about an implant?

B : He can't afford the expense of an implant.

A : Hum. How old is he?

B : Hi is 72 years old. Let me see.

I will calculate the total amount.

Eight missing teeth and one side free-end case.

There is no second molar on the opposite side which means the second molar is not required to recover.

Also he is over 70 years old which means the government insurance covers part of the payment, so the total amount will be close to a partial denture.

I will send a patient's impression today.

A : Great! If there is any change, let me know.

Also, If he doesn't like implants, then I will try to change the design of the major connector.

B : Thank you.

Chapter 8

Shopping

Key expressions

1. Shopping

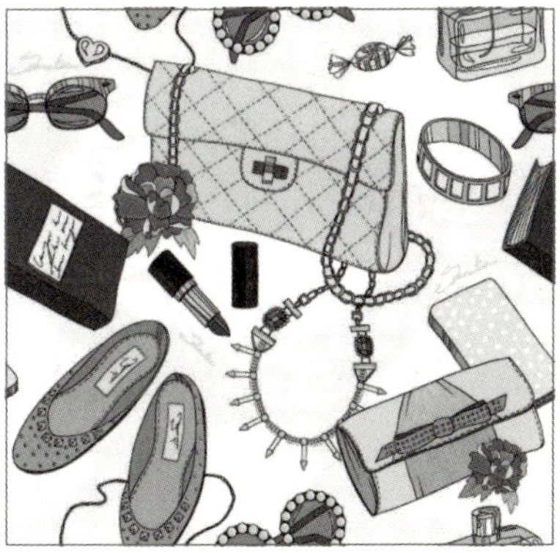

A : Can I help you?

B : I am just browsing, thanks.

A : How much is that T-shirt in the window?

B : It's 67 dollars.

A : It's too expansive. Don't you have any special offer items?

B : Oh, we're on clearance sale on second floor.

A : Oh, Great! Also, do you sell sneakers?

B : Sorry, we don't have any left.

A : I'm looking for the shampoo, too. Could you tell me where it is?

B : Yes, It's next to this shelf.

A : Do you have these trousers in stock?

B : I will check it. Yes, we have.

A : Do you know anywhere I could try?

B : Of course. Follow me please.

A : Excuse me, but what time do you close today?

B : We open 24 hours a day.

2. Payment

A : Next, please! 153 dollars, please.

B : Do you take credit card? / Can I pay by check? / I'll pay in cash.

A : Yes, you can pay it with credit.
Enter your pin, please.
Please wait.
Remove your card.
Signature, please.

B : Could I have a receipt, please?

A : OK. Would you like a bag?

B : Yes, please. And would you be able to gift wrap it for me?

A : OK. Just a moment, please.

3. Return & Complaints

A : I'd like to return this.
I'd like to refund this.
It doesn't fit. I'd like to change this for a different size.
It doesn't work.

Vocabulary

- **Browsing** : Seeing or reading superficially or at random
- **Good value** : Good price
- **In stock** : Available for use or sale
- **Pin** : A number you choose and use to gain access to various accounts
- **Signature** : Your name written in your own handwriting
- **Receipt** : An acknowledgment that payment has been made
- **Return** : Getting something back again
- **Refund** : Money returned to a payer

유용한 쇼핑용어

Special offer, clearance sale, closing down sale, buy 1 get 1 free, buy 1 get 1 half price

국소의치 제작 과정

Procedure for removable partial denture

Care of impressions and making casts

The most frequently used material for making impressions for removable partial denture is alginate and rubber base. Examine the impression to determine its acceptability. With a sharp knife, trim excess impression material extending beyond the back of the tray. Rum cold tap water gently over the impression to rinse saliva from it. Do not box an alginate impression with wax or plaster. It may dehydrate the impression, resulting in distoration. Pour the impression immediately with pre weighted stone mixed with the recommended volume of distilled water.

Custom tray

Outline the extent of the tray on the cast. Adapt the relief wax over the cast. Measure the powder and liquid according to the manufacturer's direction, and mix it. Center the plaster sheet over the cast, making sure that it covers the entire area. Before the acrylic resin tray material sets completely, some of the material may be added to the front of the tray to form a handle. After the tray material has been set, remove it from the cast. Trim the tray material with a stone or bur. When the desired length of the tray has been established, round the borders, and polish them. Male a large number of holes with a No.6 or 8 round bur.

Working cast

Wrap the boxing wax around the impression and seal the boxing wax. Vibrate a stone mix into the dry impression to form the cast. Separate the cast from the impression in 1 hour.

Survey and design

Class Ⅰ (Bilateral distal extension)

Class Ⅱ (Unilateral distal extension)

Class Ⅲ (Edentulous areas are bounded anteriorly and posteriorly by abutments)

Class Ⅳ (Anterior eduentulous)

- **Cast tilting** : Tilting is simply changing the position of the cast, which thus changes the long axis of each tooth on the cast relative to the horizontal plane.
- **Undercut** : Classified an tooth and soft tissue undercuts.
- **Preserving the tilt through tripoding** : Once a tilt has been selected, this tilt should be preserved, so it can be reestablished accurately and the cast should be removed from the survey table or the survey table should be inadvertently changed during the design procedure.

Blockout, and relief

Casts are blocked out to eliminate undercut areas on the master cast that will be crossed by rigid parts of the partial denture. Relief is used to create a space between the framework and the cast or soft tissue.

Duplication and refractory casts

The master cast must be thoroughly soaked in clear slurry water for 30 minutes. Place the cast on the base of the duplicating flask. Seat the body of the flask. Place the reservoir ring in the body. Fill the duplicating flask with agar. Cool the duplicating material in the flask. Invert the flask, and remove the base of the flask. Remove the cast. Pour the investment into the mold. Permit the investment to set for 1 hour, then separate it from the duplicating material. Place the cast in a drying oven for 2 to 3 hours. The temperature should be between 180~200°F. Immerse the cast in the bees wax.

Waxing and Spruing

Complete the framework with gauge wax and plastic patterns. Trim the cast. Attach sprue one end to the cental sprue and the other to the bottom edge of the major connector. Reinforce and smooth all junction between the sprue and the framework patterns, and they are ready for investment.

Investing, burnout, and casting

Vibrate the mix of investment and pour into casting ring. Permit the investment to set for at least 1 hour. Prepare and balance the casting machine before the casting ring is placed in the burnout oven. Place the ring in a cool furnace sprue side down. Turn the burnout furnace on and adjust it to right temperature. Wind the casting machine three or four turns and place the metal in the crucible on the asbestos liner. Light the torch, and heat the metal, keeping the tip of the blue cone on the surface of the metal. Move the arm of the casting machine to drop the locking pin. Remove investment by hand and the remaining investment with sandblaster.

Finishing and polishing the framework

Cut the sprue with a separating disk and smooth the framework except for those areas which come in contact with the teeth, such as the undersurface of occlusal rests, the minor connectors, and the inner surface of the clasp arms.

Arranging teeth

Make and position the teeth until and acceptable arrangement has been created. Mark the occlusal contact with articular ribbon and adjust using a small green stone or bur until contact is uniform. Check final occlusion.

Flasking, processing, deflasking, and finishing

Seat the cast in stone in lower half of flask. Apply stone mix to cover cast and metal framework. Do not cover wax or artificial denture teeth. Paint the stone with a separating medium. Vibrate stone mix into flask and fill it. Press top of flask in position. Place flask in boiling water and open it. Clean two halves of flask. Add powder to liquid and mix, and pack dough around and under metal. Place plastic sheet between two halves of flask and press the flask. Remove plastic sheet and close the flask. When the 1-hour bench curing time is over, place the flask in a curing unit. Remove the top of the flask with a laboratory knife. Remove stone from the denture. Remove the peripheral flash with burs or stone and finish the first stage of polishing. To avoid damaging the plastic or metal, care must be taken in using these instruments. Pumice on a wet cloth wheel should be used to remove all the scratched on the external surface of the acrylic resin.

Chapter 9

Bank

Key expressions

1. At Bank

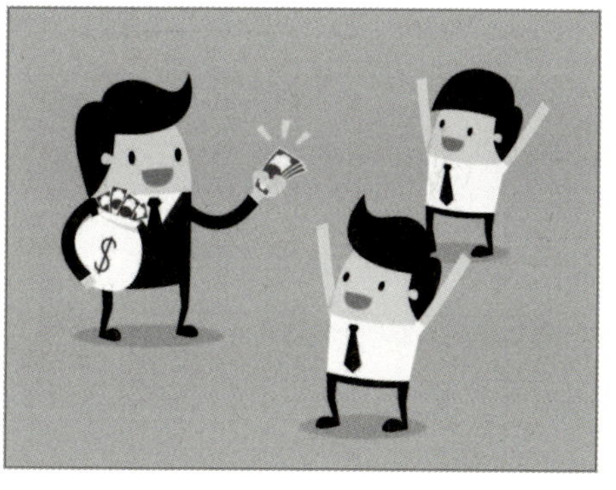

A : I'd like to open an account.

B : OK. Have you got any ID?

A : Yes, here my passport. And I'd like to pay this in, please.

B : OK. I see.

A : What's the interest rate on this account?

B : 2.7%, annually.

A : I want to make a withdrawal. 2,000 dollars, please.

B : How would you like the money?

A : In hundreds, please.

A : Could you transfer 1,000 dollars from my current account to this Korean account?

B : OK.

A : What's the exchange rate for Won?

B : The rate is 1,000 Won to the dollar.

A : Could I have a statement, please?

B : Sure.

A : I'd like to speak to someone about a mortgage(study loan/vehicle finance).

A : I've lost my bank card. / I've forgotten my banking password.

2. Make change

A : Next, please?

B : I need some change, please.

A : How do you want it?

B : Here's a $10 bill. I need 40 quarters.

A : OK. Here you are.

B : Thank you

3. Using cash machine

A : Where is the nearest cash machine(ATM)?

B : On the first floor of this building.

(At cash machine)

Insert your card

Enter your PIN.

Withdraw cash.

Please wait. Your cash is being counted.

Other service?

Would you like a receipt?

Remove card.

Incorrect PIN.

Insufficient funds

Balance

Quit

Bank Check

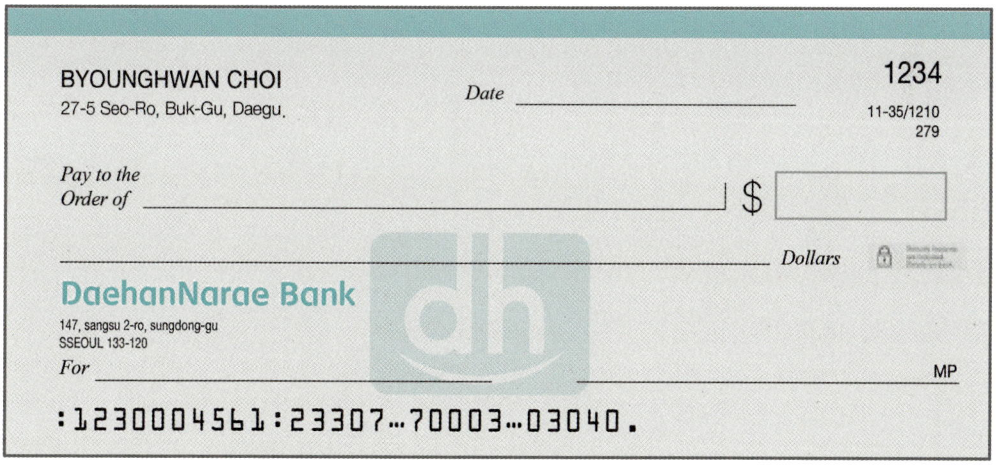
BYOUNGHWAN CHOI
27-5 Seo-Ro, Buk-Gu, Daegu.
Date
1234
11-35/1210
279
Pay to the
Order of
$
Dollars
DaehanNarae Bank
147, sangsu 2-ro, sungdong-gu
SSEOUL 133-120
For
MP
:1230004561:23307...70003...03040.

Vocabulary

- **Account** : To provide regular banking
- **ID** : Identification; something that identifies a person or thing
- **Interest** : A fixed charge for borrowing (saving) money; usually a percentage of the amount
- **Withdraw** : The act of taking out money or other capital
- **Transfer** : The act of moving money from one to another
- **Exchange** : Changing one money to another money
- **Statement** : A document showing credit and debits; a receipt
- **Insufficient** : Of a quantity not able to fulfill a need or requirement
- **Balance** : The difference between the totals of the credit and debit sides of an account

미국의 돈

미국 지폐 종류는 1, 2, 5, 10, 20, 50, 100, 500, 1,000, 5,000, 10,000, 100,000으로 분류되어 있으나 현실적으로는 100달러 이하의 권종만 사용되고 있으며, 간혹 시중에 500, 1,000달러 등의 지폐가 유통되기는 하나 그 외 고액지폐는 화폐 수집가들 외에는 소지하고 있지 않은 것으로 파악되고 있다. 미국 화폐는 전부가 동일한 크기이다.

1달러 밑으로는 센트(cent)가 존재하며, 우리나라 동전과 같은 형태로 1센트(Penny), 5센트(Nickel), 10센트(Dime), 25센트(Quarter)가 있다.

EDT : 관교의치 제작 과정

Crown & Bridge

Working Cast

Working and second cast are poured. The manufacturer's directions should be followed in regard to the water-power ratio for each stone. Mechanical spatulation, which in this case is best done under vacuum. Trim the cast and make holes, flat on one side. Set dowel pins into the abutments almost parallel to the long axes of those teeth and the ends of the dowel pins are covered with rubber caps. Fill, covering the rubber caps with different color of stone from the original. With the use of a saw, the abutment teeth are sectioned. The stone must be trimmed from the cervical margin to give access for carving the wax pattern. After being trimmed, the cast must be mounted on an articulator that can simulate the movements dictated by the occluding surfaces of the opposing teeth. The opposing cast can be related to it, using the registration.

Wax patterns

Wax patterns for restorations may be fabricated in two ways: by carving the pattern on a die(indirect method); or by carving the pattern to completion on the prepared tooth(direct method), then making the casting. In direct techniques, a Type I wax is used, whereas for indirect techniques a Type II wax is employed, the principal difference being in the amount of flow obtained at certain temperatures.

The die and working cast must be lubricated before the die is dipped into molten wax to assure a thin, contracting film next to all the prepared surfaces. Dip lubricated die into molten wax and trim to margin of preparation.

Establish contact areas, the height of contour on both buccal and lingual, the area between the clasp tios, the relation of the cusp tips to the anatomic center of the tooth as determined from the height of contour viewed from the occlusal, the relative size of the cusps, and the relation of the cusps to the marginal ridges. Correct the margins and polish the pattern.

Spruing

The size of sprue will be a determinant of the density of the casting. The sprue pin should be placed at the bulkiest part of the pattern, but not at a place where it will obliterate carving designed to promote function in lateral excursions or in centric closing. A mandibular full veneer gold crown pattern can be sprued on the lingual surface of a lingual cusp or the surface approximating an edentulous area. A maxillary crown pattern will not be damaged if the sprue pin is placed on the buccal surface of a buccal cusp. Reserviors are recommended as an aid in eliminating any inclination toward shrinkage porosity.

Investing

To compensate for the contraction of the alloy when it solidifies, three types of expansion occur in dental investment; these are setting expansion, thermal expansion, and hygroscopic expansion. The investment mold is enlarged via these three mechanisms to adjust for the shrinkage of the alloy. Use an asbestos liner to permit more freedoom in the expansion of the investment, freedom that otherwise would be restricted by the ring. It is recommended that the pattern be placed at a constant distance of 6.0mm from the open end of the ring. A liner is 3.0 or 6.0mm short of the open end of the ring. Paint a wetting agent on the surface of the pattern before investing to decrease the likelihood of enclosing air. The investment is well mixed and placed on an inside edge of the pattern with a brush. Place the ring over the painted pattern and pour the investment until the ring is filled.

Casting

Set the furnance and heat the ring(never before 30 minutes after investment). High initial burnout temperatures cause too hasty heating, with danger of cracking the mold. The heating should be slow until the free water and the water of crystallization of the plaster have been evaporated. If the temperature is increased too quickly, steam may be formed nad small piece of investment will explode off the inside of the mold, giving a rough, defective casting. Heating of the mold may be done at any suitable time.

Use approximately one-half new gold for each casting. Metal should be used in a quantity that will fill the mold and still leave an dense sprue and modest-sixed button. Remove the ring from the furnance. Melt the metal and add flux just after the metal has liquefied. This thin film of flux on the surface aids in guarding the metal against accidental oxidation during melting. In the earlier phases of the heating, the lower fusing metals liquefy while the higher fusing metals remain solid. All the alloy melts and a spheroidal mass id formed; it has a dull red color at this point. Shortly thereafter the metal becomes almost transparent and begins to spin. When the metal assume a light orange color, It is ready to cast. The casting may be a little dark, owing to surface oxidation from the investment, but it can be cleaned by pickling in a 50 per cent solution of acid. The casting should be placed in a porcelain or glass container and heated, but not boiled. The casting must be thoroughly washed in tap water. Acid may be re-used, but it should be changed regularly to mitigate any chance of contamination. A casting should never be held with steel tongs.

Polishing

A separating disk is used to cut off the sprue, and a stone and a mounted green stone are used over the cut-off sprue into the contour of casting. Q rubber wheel is used on larger surfaces. Next, a rebber point will give a satin finish to all surfaces. the occlusal and other finely carver surfaces are polished with tripoli. Every thace of rouge must be washed off.

Chapter 10

Hospital

Key expressions

1. When you are sick

(Scene 1)

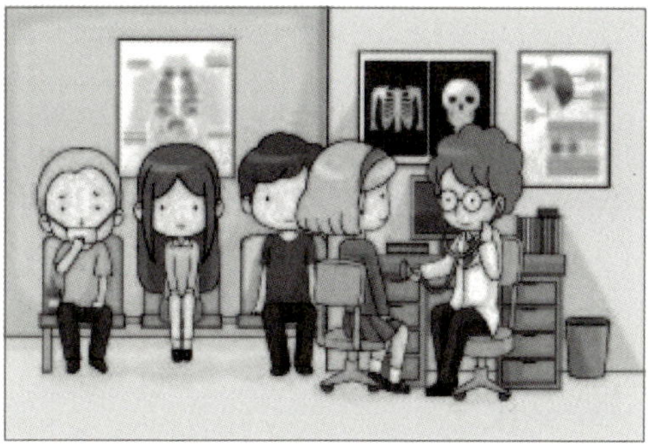

A : I'd like to see a doctor.

B : What's the problem? Is it urgent?

A : I've got a pain in my chest.

B : What are your symptoms?

A : I've got diarrhea

B : How long have you been feeling like this?

A : From yesterday.

B : Do you have any allergies?

A : No.

B : Does it hurt when I press here?

A : Oops! Yes.

B : I'm going to prescribe you some antibiotics.

Take two of these pills three times a day.

Take this prescription to the chemist.

A : OK. Thanks.

(Scene 2)

A : I am here to annual checkup.

B : How have you been feeling generally?

A : I've been feeling very hard.

B : How long have you been feeling like this?

A : I don't know exactly, but always nowadays.

B : Is there any possibility you might be pregnant?

A : Never.

B : Are you on any sort of medication?

A : Yes, I'm asthmatic

B : Can I have a look?

A : OK.

B : I'm going to take your blood pressure / temperature / pulse.

We need to take a urine sample.

(Scene 3)

A : Where does it hurt?

B : I've got a swollen ankle.

A : I want to send you for an X-ray. And I'm going to give you an injection.

2. At dentist

A : Have you had any problems?

B : I've got toothache.

A : Can you open your mouth, please?
You've got a bit of decay in this one.
Do you want to have a crown fitted?

B : Yes, please.

A : Would you like to rinse your mouth out?

B : OK.

Vocabulary

- **Symptom** : Any change in bodily function that is experienced by patient
- **DiarrheA** : Frequent and watery bowel movement
- **Prescription** : A doctor's written about medication
- **Chemist** : A health professional trained in the art of preparing drugs
- **Pregnant** : Being about to produce new life
- **Medication** : Treats or prevents the symptoms of disease; treating medicine
- **Asthmatic** : Relating to breathing with whistling sound
- **Pulse** : The rate at which the heart beats
- **Urine** : Liquid excretory product
- **Injection** : The act of putting a liquid into the body; shot
- **Decay** : Lose a stored charge
- **Crown** : The part of a tooth above the gum that is covered with enamel
- **Rinse** : Wash with clean water

도재 기공물 제작 과정

Dental ceramic

Preparation of framework (Zirconia)

Prepare the milled or sintered zirconium oxide framework with abrasive instruments. The minimum thickness of frameworks and connectors should be strictly observed. Blast the framework surface with Al_2O_3 stipulated by the manufacturer, then clean thoroughly. Apply the frame shade thinly and evenly to the zirconium oxide framework, then fire under vacuum.

Preparation of framework (PFM)

Do full wax-up and fabricate a silicone key to check the space conditions. During contouring, the thicknesses of wax frameworks are a prerequisite for the stability of the alloy frameworks. Sandblast and pickle the cast alloy frameworks and check their fit on the model. Finish the alloy frameworks using burs or grinding instruments. Blast the alloy framework with Al_2O_3 aluminium oxide. Apply the opaque in even brush strokes and fire. The second opaque firing is opaquely applied and should produce an eggshell shining. Apply separating medium and place the coping, not too tightly fitting, onto the die. To cover the shoulder use the shoulder porcelain selected for the tooth shade as far as the preparation border. After gently drying in the open firing chamber, the cap can easily be lifted off the die.

Dentin build-up

Conceals the marginal areas, pontic and interproximal using opaque dentin tooth shades to prevent shadows entering into the build-up and help color stabilization in the cervical third. Build up the labial anatomical shape of the crown with dentin porcelain. Once the anatomical form is ready, reduce the incisal and interdental areas of the dentin in order to create enough space for further layering. Irregularities are rather advantageous here. Then complete the missing areas with incisal and transparent porcelains depending on the individual appearance of the crown required. Cover the palatal surface with a darker opaque dentin. Then complete the palatal surface with incisal, transparent porcelain.

Incisal build-up

Over-contour labially and incisally to allow for firing contraction. After lifting off the model, supplement the contact points with the opaque dentin, dentin, and incisal porcelains. Separate the interdental spaces with a sharp instrument.

Dentin firing

The dentin firing takes place under vacuum. Reliable proof of a correct firing cycle can only be produced by visual checking after the firing. If the appearance is slightly shiny, the firing cycle was perfect.

Correction

Finish and clean the crowns before the correction firing. The second form firing involves making only small corrections of shape with incisal and transparent porcelains. Firing takes place under vacuum. If the firing cycle is correct, the ceramic will again appear slightly shiny.

Glaze

The crown should be finished and cleaned before glaze. Mimick discolorations on the tooth surface. Additional individual characterization can be done with suitable stains. The degree of shine of the texture can be matched to the situation in the mouth using rubber polishers, felt wheel, pumice powder and polishing tools.

Full-anatomical-contour zirconia

Zirconia can be full-anatomical-contour milled and veneered with ceramic which is minimally reducing the frame surface with bur, and then refining the surface manually with the lab hand-piece. Apply a thin layer of enamel porcelain after wash bake of various dentin shades.

Colouring

After milling framework, paint individually using a small brush which is metal-free brush in order to avoid discolourations.

Fluorescence

If so desired, milled restorations can be infiltrated with a fluorescent colour liquid prior to colouring. The fluorescence will be most visible in the incisal area.

Dry the framework under infrared lamp for at least one hour. Sinter and blast the framework with aluminium oxide. Blasting is not required on the areas to be veneered with ceramic.

Chapter 11

Hair Salon

Key expressions

1. At beauty salon

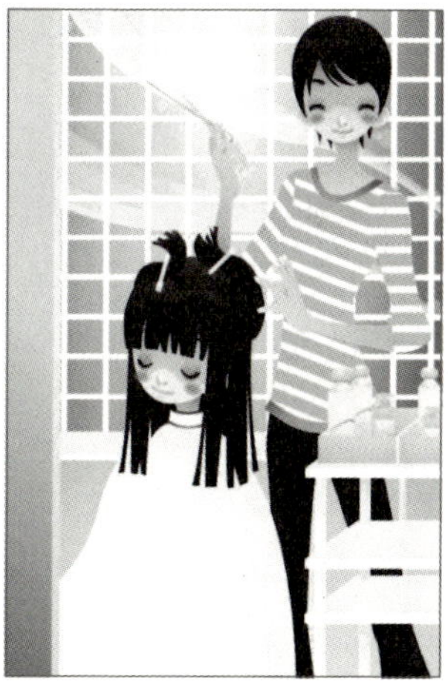

A : Are you able to see me now?
I'd like a haircut, please.
B : Yes. How would you like me to cut it?

A : Just a trim, please.
B : OK. Then, would you like it blow-dried?

A : Yes, please.
B : Do you have a parting?

A : Yes, the right side.
B : Would you like anything on it?

A : A little wax, please.

A : I'd like it colored. And I want get a perm, too.
B : Which of these colors would you like?

A : I want light brown.

B : OK. I got it. After colored, I will have your hair permed.
Do you want to tight perm or soft perm?

A : I like a soft one.

B : Would you like me to wash your hair?

A : OK. Thanks.

2. At barbers

A : Do you want to trim your beard?
Do you want to trim your moustache?

B : That's fine, thanks.

Vocabulary

- **Trim** : Cutting neat and smart
- **Blow-dried** : Blow warm air onto hair with a hand-held electric blower
- **Parting** : A line of scalp that can be seen when sections of hair are combed in opposite
- **Beard** : The hair growing on the lower part of a man's face
- **Moustache** : An unshaved growth of hair on the upper lip

기본 헤어스타일 유형

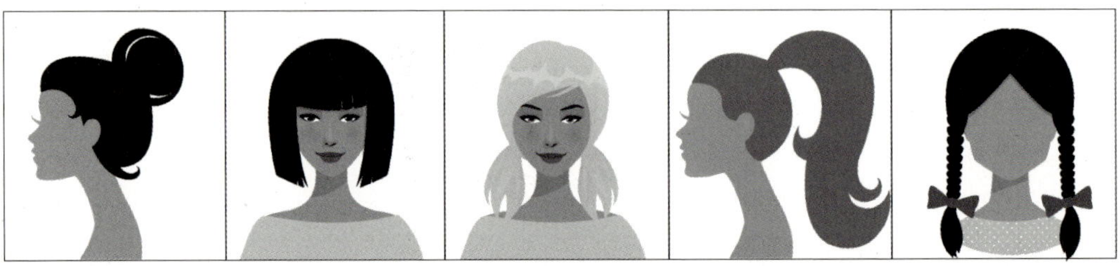

Bun　Bang　Pigtails　Ponytail　Braid

총의치 제작 과정

Complete denture

Tooth arrangement

The arrangement is influenced by age, sex, personality, and cosmetic factor. Arrangement to meet esthetic requirements is associated with the size, shape, and color of the six anterior teeth. Some of the factors influencing the size and form of the anterior teeth are the size of the face, the amount of available interarch space, the measured distance between the distal of the right and left maxillary cuspids, the length of the lips and the size and relation of the arches. The horizontal and vertical positions of the posterior teeth are involved in facial expression. The maxillary first and second bicuspids are as important to appearance as the central and lateral incisors as one sees when many people smile or laugh.

Place contoured occlusion rims on the cast, and mark the guide lines on the shoulders of the casts; midline, low lip line, cuspid line, and high lip line. Transfer the maxillary cast to the articulator with a face-bow. Mount the mandibular cast using an interocclusal wax record. Arrange the central incisor, the lateral incisor, and the cuspid on one side before the contour of the occlusion rim on the other side is removed. Arrange all the maxillary and mandibular anterior teeth reflects the symmetry of arrangement. Arrange the maxillary posterior teeth in centric occlusion with the mandibular posterior teeth. Finally, contour and smooth the wax.

Wax contouring

Countour wax carefully to prevent movement of the teeth. Avoid a bulky wax-up. Place wax along the facial surface and extend from the gingival third of the teeth to the edge of the cast. Carve the interdental palillae to resemble the natural papillae. They vary with the age of the patient. Develop the margin by carving at a 45° angle to the neck of the tooth. After the wax has been contoured, smooth it by flaming and then polish it with wet cotton.

Flasking of denture

Separate the cast from the plaster articular mounting and save the plaster mounting, as it will be used to reposition the cast on the articulator after the dentures processed. Sock the cast in the water a few minutes. Invest the lower half of the flask first. Center the cast in the lower half of the flask. Remove any undercuts in the investment. Allow the investment to set and proceed then with second investment. Apply a separating medium to the investment in the lower half of the flask. Position the ring portion of the flask and pour a mix of plaster, leaving exposed the occlusal surfaces of the posterior and the incisal edges of the anterior teeth. Apply a separating medium to the ring portion of the investment. Complete the investment with a mixture of plaster. Place the top of the flask in position, and secure the cast in the flask press.

Preparation of mold

– Wax elimination

After the flasking, let the stone copletely set; place the flask into boiling water for five minutes to soften the waxed denture base, wich can be easily removed from the mold when the flask is opened. Remove the flask from the boiling water and insert an instrument between the upper and lower halves and separate them. Remove the waxed denture base. All the teeth should remain in the top half of the flask. Flush out all the remaining wax using hot water.

Preparing and packing acrylic resin.

Measure and mix the polymer and monomer according to the manufacturer's directions. Place the lid in the jar and allow the mixture to stand; then open the jar, and test the material with a spatula. When it is doughy not sticky, the material id ready for packing. Pack the material in the upper half of the flask, press it well into the area round the teeth. Plase the cellophane over the acrylic resin. Put the loxer half of the flask in position, and press the flask together. Remove the flask from the press, open the flask and trim off the excess acrylic resin. Place the upper and lower halves of the flask in the processing press. Cure the resin in water bath at suitable temperature. After the resin of denture base has been processed, the flask should be cooled slowly to room temperature. Remove the cover and put the flask, with its open end up, into the ejector deflasking press. Cut the stone with a saw and trim the stone away.

Remount procedure

Remount the cast on the articulator so that any change in contract relation of the occlusal surfaces that may have occurred during processing may be corrected. The interceptive occlusal contacts are found by lightly tapping the teeth together on articulating paper.

Recovering the complete denture from the cast

Cut the base of the cast partly through in several directions with a saw. Insert a plaster knife into the cuts and separate the sections of stone.

Finishing and polishing the complete denture

Remove any flash of acrylic resin at the denture border, any flash and stone remaining around the teeth, surfaces of the denture base resulting from processing.

Remove all scratches and rough areas. Use a series of a mirror-like surface on the material being polished. use a brush wheel and powdered pumice to polish around the necks of the teeth and the interproximal spaces. remove the fine scratches left by the pumic with a rag wheel and tripoli, which should be used very carefully as pumice. Finally, using very light pressure, polish the denture with wet rag wheel.

Chapter 12

Traveling

1. 여행 및 호텔 (체크인, 룸서비스)

Key expressions

1. Flight reservation

A : United Airlines. May I help you?

B : I want to book my flight to L.A.

A : When do you want to?

B : On the eighth of July.

A : What's your name?

B : Hyoung-don, Jung.

A : OK. You are confirmed.

B : Thank you.

2. At hotel

1) Reservation

A : Holiday Inn. May I help you?

B : Can I make a reservation for a room?

A : Yes, sir.

B : How much is a rate?

A : 90 dollars a day.

B : I'd like to stay for two nights.

A : When will you check in?

B : I will check in August 13.

A : Do you need single room?

B : No, I want to double room.

A : What's your name?

B : My name is Yoo and first name is Jae-seok.

A : OK. Thank you for using our hotel. See you then.

2) Check-in & Check-out

A : Hello. I have reservation. My last name is Yoo.

B : Single or Double?

A : I'd like a twin bed room. How much is a rate?

B : 90 dollars a day.

A : Is that including tax?

B : No, do you have credit card?

A : Yes, I have Visa card. Here you are.

B : Could you fill this form in?

A : Sure. Is breakfast included?

B : Yes, you can use the buffet on the first floor at 7:00~10:00 in the morning.

A : And I want a room with a nice view.

B : OK. Let me see.

A : Check out, please.

B : What is your room number?

A : Twelve eighteen.

B : Here is your bill.

A : Can I pay for it in cash / traveler check?

3) During in Hotel

A : I am locked out of my room.
Can you give me a wake-up call at six thirty?

Vocabulary

- **Book** : Reserve
- **Confirm** : Strengthen or make more firm
- **Rate** : Amount of a payment; price
- **Wake-up call** : A telephone call that you request be made a specific time in order to wake you up at that time
- **Bill** : Demand payment

2. 해외 전시회

Exhibition

1. 인사

- Hello, how are you?
- Good morning, Sir or Madam? Good afternoon?
- May I help you, Sir or Madam?
- How's the exhibition?

2. 소개

- Hi, my name Colin as a sales representative / manager / director from Daegu Company.
- Please take my business card / here's my business card.
- May I have your business card? / Could I get your business card?
- My company is located in Daegu, Korea.
- Daegu Company is one of the fast growing / world leading companies in the world.
- It's good to know you, because I'd like to expand our business to your market.

3. 기본 정보 묻기

- Where do you come from? (= Where are you from?)
- Are you a dentist or a distributor?
- Are you dealing with dental equipment now?
- Which company are you cooperating now?
- If you don't mind, I'd like to introduce our product.

4. 가격 및 조건

- Our quality with reasonable / competitive price will never make you disappointed.
- How many the items can you sell in the first year?
- As you may know, the price always depends on the sales amount.
- Now all I can offer you is $50 per 1 set.
- Terms will be payment T/T in advance and FOB Korea in the first year.
- Everything can be discussed again in next year.

※ **T/T in advance** : 돈을 먼저 받고 물건을 주는 선수금 개념

In 30 days / 60 days : 흔한 할부의 개념, 제품 수령 후 30일/60일 이내 대금 지급

FOB KoreA : 구매자가 운송비를 부담하는 착불의 개념

5. 마무리

- Thank you for visiting our booth.
- Let's keep in touch!
- I will send you an email with more detailed information of our company.

3. 이메일 작성

Business email 작성 방법

제목 : Regarding/Concerning your order_0702

제목은 가장 간결하게 메일의 목적만 쓰는 것이 좋다. 뒤에 발송 당시의 날짜를 표시해 주는 것도 한 가지 팁이 될 수 있다.

◎ *Dear Mr. Lee*

가장 좋은 것은 수신자의 이름을 알고 첫머리에 써 주는 것이다. 상대방의 이름을 모를 경우 To whom it may concern (담당자 분께)/ Dear Sir or Madam 등의 표현으로 시작해도 괜찮다.

◎ *Let me start off by introducing myself. My name is Colin Lee and I am in charge of overseas sales for Daegu Company. I was referred to your address by Mr. Kim of Health Company.*

처음 발송하는 경우 이름과 직책을 먼저 밝히고, 어디서 연락처를 받았는지 언급해 주는 것이 좋다.

◎ *Daegu Company is one of the fast-growing and globally competitive Dental Lab located in Daegu, Korea. We are now selling our products in more than 10 countries, but have had no connection in your market yet.*

Since these days it is important to make people think of dental treatment *not as an expensive luxury, but as a standard quality-of-care option, Daegu Company would be the best solution for you.*

본문의 내용이 너무 길 경우 상대방도 읽기 힘들고, 착오가 생길 수 있기 때문에 요점만 간략히 적어 주는 것이 좋다.

◎ *I would like to establish a good partnership with you / I look forward to hearing from you soon.*

마무리 인사

◎ *Sincerely (= Faithfully / Wishes / Kind Regards / All the best)*

Colin. (이름)

위의 표현을 사용하여 끝맺음을 한다.

4. 기초 무역 용어

① PO(Purchase Order) : 주문서(수입업체에서 주문을 줄 때 사용)

② PI(Proforma Invoice) : 견적 송장(수출업체가 받은 주문에 대한 견적서)

③ CI(Commercial Invoice) : 상업 송장(주문에 대한 확정 후 발행되는 최종 invoice)

④ PL(Packing List) : 포장 명세서(선적을 위해 포장된 물품에 대한 디테일)

⑤ BL(Bill of Lading) : 선하증권, 운송화물의 수령 또는 선적을 인증하는 서류. 우리나라 택배 운송장과 비슷한 개념

⑥ Courier : FEDEX, DHL, TNT 같은 국제 배송업체를 이용해 물품을 발송하는 것

⑦ Forwarding : Courier가 아닌 일반 운송업체를 통해 물품 발송하는 것. Courier보다 저렴하지만 배송 기간이 오래 걸림

⑧ Incoterms : 무역 거래에 있어 물품의 판매 가격을 결정할 때 사용하는 정형화된 국제 표기 방법

⑨ Clearance : 통관

⑩ Customs Duties : 관세

memo

Chapter 13

Go Around

1. 길 찾기 및 교통 이용

Key expressions

1. Way-finding

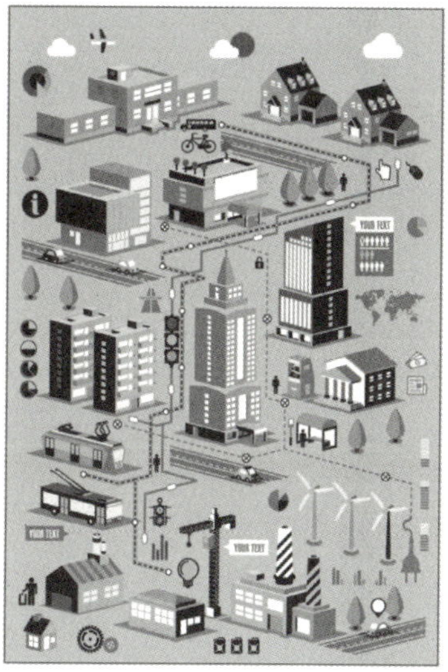

A : Do you know where 16141 Hereon Ave. is?

B : Keep on going this way about one hundred meters.

And you will see a ten-story white building on the same side.

Turn left at the building. And Go straight up.

Turn right on the third crossing.

Then you will see a red brick house ahead of you.

A : Oh, It's complicate.

B : Let me draw a map for you.

A : OK. Thanks. How long does it take to get there on foot?

B : Not so far. It takes about 20 minutes, I guess.

A : Thank you for your kindness.

B : It's my pleasure.

2. Using Transportation

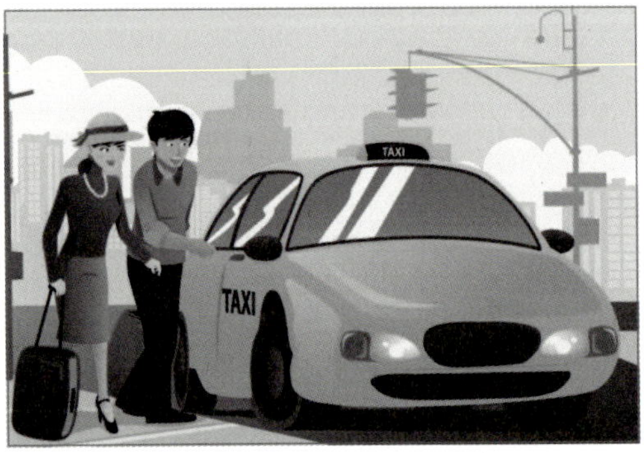

1) Taxi

A : Where is the nearest taxi stand?

B : Cross the road.

(take a taxi)

A : Where to sir?

B : To the airport, please. / Take me to this address, please.

A : Would you put my bag in the truck?

B : Sure.

A : How much will it be to airport?

B : May be 50 dollars.

(arrive to the airport)

A : OK. Stop here please. How much?

B : 49.50 dollars, please.

2) Bus

A : Is there a bus to Central station?

How often does this bus run?

Where can I get the timetable for the bus?

Where can I get a bus ticket?

How much is it to Central station?

Is this bus going to Central station?

Could you tell me when we get there?

3) Subway

A : How can I get to the subway station?

Where can I take the green line?

Which line goes to Statue of Liberty?

Which line should I change to?

When is the last subway?

If I want to get to City Hall, which exit should I take?

A : Where is the ticket booth?

Are vending machines available?

Can I get this card recharged?

Vocabulary

- **Brick** : Rectangular block of clay baked; used as a building
- **Complicate** : Make more complex
- **Vending machines** : A machine for selling goods
- **Recharge** : Charge anew

2. 해외 마케팅

Dialogue : Business

(A : Sales Manager / B : Dealer)

A : Good morning, how may I help you, sir?

B : Hi, good morning.

I'm actually looking for a manufacturer who can offer me a dental implant.

A : If so, you've come to right place because Daegu Company is one of the fastest growing manufacturers of dental implants and instruments in South Korea.

Where do you come from?

B : My name is Mohamed from Iran and I am working for the Iran Dental Company as a marketing director.

Do you have any distributors in Iran?

A : We've tried to have connections in Iran, but have not yet found a suitable partner.

So, if you are interested in doing business with Daegu Company, there's no problem.

B : It sounds perfect.

Are you selling the product in any other Middle East countries right now? Like Turkey, UAE, Syria or somewhere else?

A : Of course, we have distributors in Turkey, Iraq and Jordan.

Also we are doing very well in some European countries like France, Germany and Spain as well.

B : By the way, in how many countries are you selling the products?

A : More than 20 countries at this moment.

B : Good. Do you have your catalogues here?

A : Sure, this is the catalog of our main product named the D-Implant.
Also have a look at our actual product there. If you want, I will give you some samples.

B : Thanks. Could you please quote me prices for orders of one hundred unit of D-Implant?

A : If you make an order of one hundred of D-Implant, it could be $50 per each implant.

B : Wait, is there a MOQ for D-Implant?

A : Actually not. But we recommend you to buy a unit of 100 implants.

B : I see, what about the payment and shipping method?
Could you give me credit?

A : Unfortunately, we don't allow credit at the beginning.
But after some time like maybe 6 months or 1 year, we can discuss it again and normally we give credit of 30 or 60 days for our old and reliable partner.
And every shipping method would be possible, but courier services like DHL, FedEx or TNT are recommended.

B : Okay, I understand then. Anyway can I get your business card?
I will contact you also via email once I get back to my office.

A : Sure, please take it. Can I take yours as well?

B : No problem. Thank you for your time and keep in touch.

A : I hope we speak again very soon. Take care.

3. 견적 송장, 주문서

P/O (Purchase Order)

흔히 말하는 주문서로, 수입업체가 수출업체에게 물건을 주문할 때 사용한다. 업체 내부적으로 일정하게 정해진 양식을 사용하기도 하지만, 흔히 Email, Skype, 일반 유선전화 등으로 주문하는 경우에도 PO로 본다. 일반적으로는 General term and condition은 생략되고, 품목, 수량, 가격, 결제 조건, 선적 조건이 포함되어 있다.

- Sample

Order Info.	P.O no.	PO-1082014-01	Purchase Order
	Customer	OO Company	
	Order Date	July 24th, 2014	
	Request Date	August 24th, 2014	

No.	Ref. Code	Description	Q'ty	U/P	Amount	Remark
1	DD1	D-Implant	10	$50.00	$500.00	
2	DD2	D-Implant	10	$50.00	$500.00	
3	DD3	D-Implant	10	$50.00	$500.00	
4	DD4	D-Implant	10	$50.00	$500.00	
5	DD5	D-Implant	10	$50.00	$500.00	
6	DD6	D-Implant	10	$50.00	$500.00	
7	DD7	D-Implant	10	$50.00	$500.00	
8	DD8	D-Implant	10	$50.00	$500.00	
9	DD9	D-Implant	10	$50.00	$500.00	
10	DD10	D-Implant	10	$50.00	$500.00	
11	DD11	D-Implant	10	$50.00	$500.00	
12	DD12	D-Implant	10	$50.00	$500.00	
	TOTAL		120		$6,000.00	

P/I (Proforma Invoice)

견적 송장이라 하고, 실제 거래된 물품이 아닌, 주문 받은 물품의 가격을 견적해 주는 송장을 뜻한다. 품목, 수량, 가격 및 general term and condition이 포함되어 있고, 대금 결제 시 사용 되기도 한다.

Sample

PROFORMA INVOICE

Date : 21th Jul. 2015

1. Recipient :
2. Proforma Invoice no.: 3. Ref. P.O. no.:
4. Description :

No.	Ref. Code	Description	Q'ty	Unit Price	Amount
1		D-Implant	100	US$50	US$5,000
		TOTAL	100		US$5,000

5. Incoterm's :
6. Terms of Payment : 60 Days after shipment
7. Destination :
8. Shipping Method : Airway
9. Inspection : Standard inspection by manufacturer
10. Packing : Standard export packing
11. Remark :
    Bank Name :
    Bank Address :
    Amount No. :
    Swift :
    Beneficiary :

Authorized Signature

By

Typed Name :
Title :

By

Typed Name :
Title :

C/I (Commercial Invoice)

상업 송장이라 하고 실제 거래된 물품에 대한 송장이다. 계산서, 명세서, 대금청구서 등의 역할을 하며, 분할 선적될 경우 1개의 PO당 여러 개의 CI가 존재할 수 있다.

Sample

<table>
<tr><th colspan="6">COMMERCIAL INVOICE</th></tr>
<tr><td colspan="3" rowspan="2">(1) Seller</td><td colspan="3">(7) Invoice No. and date</td></tr>
<tr><td colspan="3">(8) L/C No. and date</td></tr>
<tr><td colspan="3">(2) Consignee</td><td colspan="3">(9) Notify party (if other than consignee)</td></tr>
<tr><td colspan="3">(3) Departure date :</td><td colspan="3" rowspan="2">(10) Other references</td></tr>
<tr><td colspan="3">(4) Vessel/Flight :</td></tr>
<tr><td colspan="3">(5) from :</td><td colspan="3" rowspan="2">(11) Terms of delivery and payment</td></tr>
<tr><td colspan="3">(6) To :</td></tr>
<tr><td>(12) HS-CODE</td><td>(13) Product code</td><td>(14) Goods description</td><td>(15) Q'ty</td><td>(16) U/Price</td><td>(17) Amount</td></tr>
<tr><td colspan="3">TOTAL</td><td colspan="2">0</td><td>US$</td></tr>
<tr><td colspan="6">Authorized Signature

By

Typed Name :
Title :

By

Typed Name :
Title :</td></tr>
</table>

The terminology of dental technology

A

abrasive paste
absorption
abutment
acid etching
acrylic resin
acrylic resin veneer
adhesion.
adjustment
agar
alginate
align
anatomic crown
anterior teeth
antiseptic
arch
arrangement
articulating paper
articulator
artificial stone
asbestos
autogenous glaze
autopolymerizing resin
axial

B

backing
base metal
baseplate
bicuspid or premolar
boiling point
bolus
bruxism
burn out
burnish
butt joint

C

cameo surface
cantilever fixed partial denture
caries
carnauba wax
centigrade
centrifugal
centripetal
ceresin
cervix
characterization
chewing cycle

chroma
chuck
clinical crown
closed bite
coalescence
cohesion.
cold cure
cold flow
collar
compensating curve
compression molding
concave
condensation
conductivity
condyle
congenital
convex
cope
coronal
creep
crest of the ridge
crystallization
cyanoacrylate

D

dappen dish
debubblizer
decalcification
deciduous tooth.
decreased occlusal vertical dimension
dentition
dentulous
deoxidizing
desiccate
devitrification
diagnosis
diagnostic cast
diastema
diatoric
disclude
disinfectant
dough
dowel
drag
ductility

E

eccentric
edentulous
electroplating
electropolishing
elongation
emergence profile
emery
eminence
endodontia
etiology
eugenol
excursion
external or lateral

extracoronal
extraoral
extrinsic
extrinsic coloring
extrusion

F

facial moulage
facing
festooningl
fin.
fistula
flange
flash
flat plane tooth
fox plate
freeway space
fusible
fusion temperature

G

garnet
gelatin
gingivectomy
gingivitis

H

heat soaking
heel of a denture
height of contour
high lip line
hue
humidor
hydration
hydrocal
hygienic pontic
hyperplasia
hyperplastic tissue

I

incisive foramen
inclination
index
induction current
inferior
initial set
intaglio surface
interarch distance
intercondylar distance
interdigitation
interim prosthesis
interlock
intermaxillary space
internal or medial
interocclusal rest space
intraoral tracing
intrinsic coloring

L

lamina dura

lateral interocclusal record
laterotrusion
ledging
lesion
leverage

M
malleability
malocclusion
malposition
mandibular
masseter muscle
master cast
mastication
masticatory cycle
matrix
maximum intercuspation (MI)
metamerism
modulus of elasticity

N
nonworking side occlusal contacts

O
oblique ridge
orbitale
orientation of occlusal plane
ovoid arch form
oxypropane torch

P
pantograph
passivity
pathogen
pathogenic
patrix
pennyweight
periapical
periodontics
periodontium
peripheral roll
petrolatum.
phonation
phonetics
pier abutment
pigment
pit
placement
porosity
porous
postpalatal seal
preliminary cast
preliminary impression
prognosis
propane
prophylaxis
proportional limit
prosthesis
prosthodontics
protrude

protrusion
protrusive articulation
protrusive interocclusal record

Q

quadrant
quench

R

reciprocity
reinforced acrylic pontic(RAP)
resorption
rest seat preparation
retention of a clasp
reverse articulation
ridge relationship
ridge resorption

S

safeside disk
sagittal plane
sanitary pontic.
sanitization
semirigid fixed partial denture
serrated
shelf life
shellac base
sideshift
slurry
soft palate
soluble
solute
solvent
sprue former
stent
sterilization
stone core
strut
sulcus
supernumerary tooth
suture line
swage
symphysis

T

tang
template
torque.
torus
translatory (sliding) motion
transverse horizontal axis
transverse plane
transverse ridge
trapezoid
trauma
treatment partial.
trifurcated
tube tooth
tubercule
tuberosity

V

vault

vibrating line

vitrification

volatile

volatility

vomer

W

warpage

weld

X

xerostomia

저 자

최 병 환 (대구보건대학교 치기공과)

박 미 영 (이화여자대학교 영어영문학과)

감 수

James Parr (대구보건대학교 교양학부)

Practical English *for* Dental Technology 2nd edition

발행일	2015년 9월 5일
저 자	최 병 환·박 미 영
발행인	최 용 원
편 집	장 순 임
표 지	장 순 임
발행처	**대한나래출판사**
등 록	제2012-000051호(1994.6.10)
주 소	서울특별시 성동구 성수2로 147 (성수동2가 289-319번지) 아이에스비즈타워 903호
전 화	(02) 922-7080
팩 스	(02) 922-0841
이메일	nrpub@naver.com

ISBN 978-89-5741-414-9 **정가 18,000원**

* 파본은 교환해 드립니다. **www.dhpub.com**